Pharmacology

(For Pharmacy)

Dr. Vivek Bele

M.D.

CAREER

Publications

Pharmacology
(For Pharmacy)

FIRST EDITION : DECEMBER 2001
FIRST EDITION REPRINT : FEBRUARY 2005
FIRST EDITION REPRINT : JULY 2006
FIRST EDITION REPRINT : AUGUST 2008

ISBN : 978-81-88739-09-7

Published by :
Nishad Deshmukh
Career Publications
Reg. Off. : 432/B, Deshmukh Bungalow ,
Vakil Wadi, Nashik - 422 001.
Maharashtra, India

Communication Address :
First Floor, Kaveri Smruti, Vakil Wadi,
Ashok Stambh, Nashik - 422001
Maharashtra, India.
Ph. : (0253) 2311422, 2576175
E-mail : publications@careerandyou.com
www.careerandyou.com

Pune Office :
First Floor, Gokhale
Classes Bldg., Tilak Road,
Pune - 411 030.
Maharashtra, India.
Ph. : (020) 24497602

Typesetting :
Career Publications, Nashik

Printer :
Replica Printers, Nashik

Price : Rs. 200/-

PREFACE

Dear friends,

This book is not meant for those who want to learn pharmacology in details.

Pharmacology is a strange subject. Sudden overexposure to this subject creates a chaos and produces long lasting disinterest. That is the reason why pharmacology is always blamed as a subject for 'memory exercise'.

Memory is an essential tool in learning pharmacology. But unfortunately human brain has limited number of neurons. They definitely are not sufficient if one decides to depend only on memory. The primary motive behind writing this book is to reduce contribution of memory while learning pharmacology. Conceptual clarity creates interest and interesting things are easily remembered.

There are lots of good books on pharmacology, which discus pharmacology in details. This book is designed to facilitate simple and uncomplicated introduction to undergraduate pharmacology students. That is the reason why content is restricted. Otherwise adding a few hundred pages is not a difficult task. All possible care has been taken to avoid mistakes, especially regarding doses of drugs. But there are always varieties of limitations on this front. I am sorry for unnoticed mistakes.

Though it seems formal, I must thank a few people. First of all I would like here to express gratitude to Dr. Pandit and Dr. Nandal for introducing me to the subject of pharmacology. My thanks are due to Dr. Shashank Shrotriya for his chapter on cardiac arrhythmia.

I am grateful to Mr.Suryawanshi for his support in making the language simple and correct.

I must appreciate Career publication for offering me a complete freedom. There can be a debate on the issue, who has worked harder for this book, Mukesh or myself.

This book would not have been written without Shilpa.

Vivek Bele.

This is a *'book and notebook'* of pharmacology.

The space is provided, on each page, with two intentions in mind:

A few things that are printed here, you can't afford to forget.

The blank space is provided for additional material, which you can collect from any other book or lectures.

In a way, this can serve as a book and a notebook.

OUR EARLIER PUBLICATIONS

For B. Pharm

1)	Career in Pharmacy : Thoughts & Views	:	Milind Wagh
2)	Inorganic Pharmaceutical Chemistry (Theory)	:	Dr. Tipnis & Dr. Dhake
3)	Inorganic Pharmaceutical Chemistry (Practical)	:	Dr. Belsare & Dr. Dhake
4)	Anatomy Physiology and Health Education	:	Rahul Phate
5)	Experimental Pharmaceutical Organic Chemistry - A Benchtop Manual	:	K.S. Jain, P.B. Miniyar, & T.S. Chitre
6)	Modern Dispensing Pharmacy	:	Dr. A. P. Pawar & Dr. R. S.Gaud
7)	Practical Physical Pharmacy	:	H.N. More & A.A. Hajare
8)	Pharmaceutical Microbiology-Experiments and Techniques	:	Dr. C. R. Kokare
9)	Biostatistics	:	Dr. Sai Subramanian
10)	Pathophysiology for Pharmacy	:	Dr. Prakash Ghadi
11)	Introduction to Clinical Biochemistry	:	Dr. (Mrs.) Dandekar
12)	Pharmaceutical Analysis - I (Practical)	:	Sonali Sheorey & Meera Honrao
13)	Pharmacology for Pharmacy	:	Dr. Vivek Bele
14)	A Handbook of Experiments in Pre-clinical Pharmacology	:	Dr. Sanjay B. Kasture
15)	Pharmacognosy & Phytochemistry Part - I	:	Dr. Vinod Rangari
16)	Pharmacognosy & Phytochemistry Part -II	:	Dr. Vinod Rangari
17)	Principles & Applications of Biopharmaceutics and Pharmacokinetics	:	Dr. Tipnis & Dr. Amrita Bajaj
18)	Business Accounting	:	Dr. Mahesh Kulkarni
19)	Managerial Economics	:	Prof. Geet, Prof. Morajkar, Milind Wagh
20)	Industrial Psychology and Sociology	:	Milind Wagh

For D. Pharm

1)	Human Anatomy & Physiology	:	Rahul Phate
2)	Text Book of Biochemistry & Clinical Pathology	:	M. J. Umekar, R. H. Lohiya, N. R. Kotagale,
3)	Theory and Practice Pharmaceutics - I	:	Dr. A.P. Pawar
4)	Theory and Practice Pharmaceutics - II	:	Dr. A.P. Pawar
5)	Pharmaceutical Chemistry II	:	Dr. A.S. Dhake
6)	Handbook for Community Pharmacists (Exclusively for Chemists and Druggists)	:	Dr. A.P. Pawar
7)	Introduction to Pharmaceutical Chemistry	:	S.K. Banerjee, Dr. Rajashree Mashru, Dr. Gayatri Banerjee

Reference Books ....

1)	Clinical Pharmacy	:	Dr. Tipnis & Dr. Amrita Bajaj
2)	Hospital Pharmacy	:	Dr. Tipnis & Dr. Amrita Bajaj

For GATE Study ....

1)	GATE : A Companion (for pharmacy)	:	N.N.Inamdar
2)	Pharmacy GATE Solved Question Papers (1988-2006)	:	N.N.Inamdar
3)	Career GATE Postal Test Series	:	For details write to us

Foreign Titles

1)	Lexi-com's Pharmacogenomics Handbook	:	Cavallari, Ellingrod & Kolesar

CONTENTS

* * *

GENERAL PHARMACOLOGY

"THIS SECTION CONTAINS"

Definition of Drug

World Health Organization defines drug as any substance or product that is used or intended to be used to modify or explore physiological system or pathological state for the benefit of the recipient. The term medicine includes, in addition to drug, the substances used to deliver drug in stable and acceptable form.

Pharmacology

It is the science that deals with the origin, nature, chemistry, effects and uses of drugs. In brief, it is a study of drugs.

Sources of drugs

Drugs are obtained from different sources. Most of the drugs that are currently used are manufactured synthetically. (Refer Table 1.1)

Table No. 1.1 Sources of Drugs.

Source	Specific source & Drugs	Category
Plants	Belladonna alkaloids: Atropine Foxglove: Digitalis	Anticholinergic Cardiac glycoside
Microbes	Penicillium Notatum: Penicillin Actinomycetes: Streptomycin E Coli: L-asparaginase	Antibiotic Antibiotic Anticancer
Animal	Pork, Beef: Insulin Horse: Tetanus antitoxin Various animals: Heparin	Antidiabetic Antitetanus Anticoagulant
Minerals	Gold Magnesium sulfate Aluminium hydroxide	Antiarthritic Purgative Antacid
Synthetic	Aspirin, Cimetidine	Antiinflammatory Acid reducing agent

Recently, drugs are synthesized by genetic technologies like human recombinant gene technology. Ex. Erythropoetin

Different ways of using drugs

In clinical practice drugs are used for different therapeutic advantages.

Curative use

In this situation drugs remove the cause of disease and eliminate disease. Ex. Antibiotics kill organisms and remove the cause of infections.

Suppressive or symptomatic uses of the drugs

In this situation drugs do not cure disease but suppress symptoms and provide temporary relief. Ex. Analgesic agents relieve pain in arthritis but do not cure the disease or cough suppressants reduce cough in respiratory infections but do not kill microorganisms.

Prophylactic or Preventive use of drugs

There are situations in which drugs are administered to prevent a specific pathological condition. In primary prevention, the individual does not have any pathology. Ex. Any vaccination. In secondary prevention, patient has some underlying pathology and to avoid the complications, preventive administration of drug is required. Ex. Aspirin prevents aggregation of platelets and reduces chances of formation of clot. Therefore it is used as antiplatelet agent for cardiac patients to prevent attacks of myocardial infarction.

Diagnostic uses of drugs

This type of application of drug offers neither cure nor symptomatic relief but it can help in diagnosis of the underlying pathology. Ex. Barium. This is a radioactive substance and is visible in x-ray films. After taking it by oral or rectal route, serial x-rays of GI tract are taken. Accumulation of barium at some point in the tract indicates obstruction while leakage indicates perforation.

Auxiliary use of drugs

In this type of use, two drugs are administered together. One drug supports the action of the other. Supporting drug does not have direct action on the disorder. Ex. When penicillin and probenecid are given together, penicillin kills organisms and probenecid reduces the renal elimination of penicillin and prolongs its action. Probenecid has no action on microorganisms.

Placebo

Literary meaning of this Latin word is 'I shall be pleasing or acceptable'. This actually is a dummy medication. If a drug has no specific biological activity for the condition being treated the drug is termed as placebo. Such drugs provide psychological relief to the patient. This type of treatment is mainly useful in mild psychological disorders or painful conditions when diagnosis of disease is in doubt.

What happens to a drug when it enters into body ?

To simplify various terms in pharmacological interactions between drug and body, let us discuss one example. Suppose a person takes 1 ml intramuscular injection to reduce his heart rate. After injection into muscles, the drug goes from muscle into the blood vessels around muscles. Blood contains some proteins that are called plasma proteins. A part of that drug gets attached to these proteins and a part remains free. The drug, during the circulation, goes to various organs in the body. When it goes to heart, it reduces the heart rate. When it goes to other organs, it may produce some undesired effects, say headache. This reduction in heart rate or headache is taken as interference in body function. When drug produces any interference in the body functions, body treats that drug as a foreign body (even though we take it for benefit of body). Body always tries to get rid of that drug. Therefore it converts that drug into a form that can be removed out of body easily. After this

Curative: to remove cause

Suppressive: for temporary relief

Diagnostic: for diagnosis

Prophylactic: for prevention

Auxiliary: supportive

Placebo: psychological advantage

Body treats drug as a foreign body

conversion, the drug is converted into an excretable form. Many times drug also is converted into inactive form to terminate the action of the drug and finally the drug is eliminated from the body. This is the journey and fate of a drug in human body. Though this journey is presented serially, actually this is a simultaneous and continuous process. Now refer to Figure 1.1. The figure expresses same process with scientific terminologies.

Figure 1.1 What happens to a drug in human body

Intramuscular injection of a drug	← Administration.
↓	
Drug in muscles.	
↓	
Drug in blood.	← Absorption.
↓	
Some part of the drug is attached to proteins and some part is free	
↓	
Drug goes in various compartments in the body	← Distribution
↓	
Desired Effects	← Actions
Undesired Effects	← Adverse actions
↓	
Conversion of drug into an excretable form	← Biotransformation or metabolism
↓	
Removal of the drug	← Excretion or elimination

Though this discussion is in reference to intramuscular injection, it holds true for all routes (with some exceptions which are discussed later).

Now let us define these terms -

Administration: It is the introduction of a drug into human body.

Absorption: It is a transfer of a drug from the site of administration into circulation.

Distribution: It is the transfer of a drug from circulation into various compartments of the body.

Desired effects: These are the effects produced by drugs for which the drug is administered.

Undesired effects: These are the effects that are produced as by-products of drugs. Most of the times they are harmful. Sometimes undesired effects are used therapeutically. Ex. Minodixil, a vasodilator produced 'hair growth' as undesired effect, which now is used as therapeutic effect.

Biotransformation or Metabolism: It is the conversion of drugs into a form that gets excreted easily. i.e.water soluble form.

Excretion or elimination: Removal of a drug from body.

After entry of a drug into human body there is a continuous interaction between drug and body. The drug does something to the body and body does a few things to that drug.

Pharmacokinetics is the term designated to what a body does to a drug and pharmacodynamics means what a drug does to a body.

Pharmacokinetics includes: Absorption, Distribution, Metabolism, and Excretion

The terms that are defined in relation to the fate of drug in the body can be classified either in pharmacokinetics or pharmacodynamics.
As the interaction of drug and body starts after the administration, administration is neither included in pharmacokinetics nor in dynamics.

Pharmacodynamics includes: Desired and undesired effects

Absorption	Body absorbs the drug	Pharmacokinetics
Distribution	Body distributes the drug	Pharmacokinetics
Desired effects	Drug produces desired effects	Pharmacodynamics
Undesired effects	Drug produces undesired effects	Pharmacodynamics
Biotransformation	Body converts drug into excretable form	Pharmacokinetics
Excretion	Body removes the drug	Pharmacokinetics

In brief, pharmacokinetics means what a body does to a drug and it includes absorption, distribution, biotransformation and excretion. Pharmacodynamics is what a drug does to a body and it includes desired and undesired effects that are produced by drugs.

Drug administration

Under the heading '*administration*', Drug nomenclature, Drug formulations, Expression of a dose of a drug and various routes of administration are included. In the discussion, various formulations are not covered to avoid encroachment over pharmaceutics. The routes of administration are discussed later because to compare various routes one must understand a few things which are discussed in the later part of this section.

DRUG NOMENCLATURE

It is a science of giving names to drugs. Drugs are titled by three different types of names.

i) Chemical Name:

It is the name of the drug that expresses chemical nature of the drug. For example, 1 - (isopropylamino) - 3 - (1' - napthyloxy) propan - 2 - ol is the chemical name for propranolol.

ii) Generic or Nonproprietary Name

Complex chemical names are not suitable for day to day use and for prescription purpose. Standard official names are used to express the chemical names. These names are accepted and approved by various scientific bodies including WHO. Diazepam, Ranitidine etc. are the examples of generic names. Generic name is not a property of any pharmaceutical companies. Sometimes generic names are approved for drug combinations. Ex. Co-amoxiclav is the generic name for the combination of amoxycillin and clavulanic acid, co-trimoxazole is the combination of trimethoprim and sulphamethoxazole.

Chemical and Generic names are universal. Brand name is specific for particular company

iii) Proprietary or Brand Name:

It is a specific name assigned to a formulation of generic drug by a specific company. It is the property or trade mark of that company. Ex. For the generic name diazepam, one company's proprietary name is 'Calmpose' whereas 'Valium' is the proprietary name of another company. Doctors are supposed to write brand names in prescriptions.

Medical practitioners should prefer proprietary or brand names in prescription

PRESCRIPTION

Prescription is a document prepared by a medical practitioner. It describes details of the medications that are to be issued to the patient. It ensures accuracy, safety and prevents misuse of drugs. An ideal prescription contains.

- Date
- Name and address of the doctor
- Name, age, sex and address of the patient.
- ℞ The sign is a symbol for Egyptian sun god and means Recipe
- Name of the drug : Doctors are supposed to write formulation and to prefer brand names of drugs.
- Amount of the drug per dose
- Frequency of administration. This specifies how many times patient is advised to take the medication.
- Duration of treatment : It specifies the number of days for which patient will take the medication.
- Route of administration
- Signature of doctor

Model prescription

Date :xxxxxx

Name and address of doctor xxxxxx

Name, age, sex and address of patient xxxxx.

℞

Tab. AMOX 500 mg. orally three times a day for 5 days.

Signature of doctor: xxxxx

Abbreviations to express the frequency of dosage administration

OD: once a day, **BD (bid):** twice a day, **TDS (TID):** thrice a day, **QDS (QID):** four times a day, **HS (on):** every night, **om:** every morning **ac:** before food **pc:** after food, **SOS:** if necessary.

Passage of drug across cell membrane

Drug, in the body, gets transferred into various compartments of the body (viz. from intestine to blood, from blood to various organs, back into blood, from blood to liver, from kidneys to urine etc.). All these movements involve passage of drug across some membranes like cell membrane of mucosal cells of digestive tract or cell membrane of capillaries, etc. All these membranes are called as biological membranes.

Structure of biological membrane

These membranes of living cell in human body are permeable interface between cell and its environment. It is a lipid bilayer in the fluid form with glycoproteins. Proteins in the cell membrane either freely float through the membrane or some of them extend through full thickness of the membrane and provide pores. Some proteins function as enzymes while some as carriers.

Drugs are transported across various body cell membranes by different mechanisms.

Mechanisms of drug transport

- Passive diffusion
- Filtration
- Carrier mediated transport
  - Active
  - Facilitated
- Pinocytosis

PASSIVE DIFFUSION

It is the most important and common mode of transport of drugs. As the name suggests, it is passive process that does not require cellular energy. Drug is passively transported according to concentration gradient (i.e. from high concentration to low concentration) from one compartment to another through cell membranes. Rate of passive diffusion depends upon two factors.

a) Ionization status of drugs or lipid solubility.

b) Concentration gradient.

Passive diffusion doesn't require energy

a) <u>Ionization status</u>: Ionized form is a charged form of a drug. Depending on ionization status, drugs are classified as:

i) Some drugs are permanently in unionized form (in body) and the status is not altered by environment in the body.

ii) Some drugs are permanently in ionized form (in body) and the status is not altered by environment in the body.

iii) In some drugs, ionization status is altered by environmental pH.

Cell membranes are mainly formed of lipids. Unionized form of a drug is a lipid soluble form and hence transfer is faster for that form. Ionized form is not lipid soluble or it is water soluble, so the transport of such drugs through membrane is slow.

Drugs in unionized form are lipid soluble and their diffusion is fast.

Drugs that are permanently in unionized form are called as lipid soluble drugs and diffusion is faster for them. Drugs that are permanently in ionized form are water soluble drugs and diffusion is slower. For drugs whose ionization status is variable, diffusion rate depends on the pH of the external environment.

Drugs in ionized form are water-soluble and slowly diffused.

Acidic drugs are not ionized in acidic medium. In other words, they remain in unionized or lipid soluble form and get diffused easily. Similarly alkaline drugs are diffused faster in alkaline medium.

Acidic drugs are transported better in acidic medium while basic drugs in basic medium.

Acidic drugs are ionized in alkaline medium and become water soluble. Hence, diffusion is slow. Similarly diffusion of alkaline drugs is slow in acidic medium.

Clinical implication:

a) Aspirin is acidic in nature and its ionization status is altered by change in pH. In stomach pH is acidic therefore aspirin is in unionized form and gets rapidly diffused from GI cavity to mucosal cells. The cellular pH is basic and aspirin gets converted into ionized form. This prevents transport of aspirin from these cells and it is accumulated in GI cells.

b) Concentration gradient: The term expresses the concentration difference between two compartments. Obviously the diffusion rate is directly proportional to concentration gradient. Amount of drug that is administered governs concentration gradient.

FILTRATION

Adjacent cells in cell membrane are joined to each other by tight junctions. Filtration is the passage of drugs through pores between two cells and the transfer is according to the osmotic gradient. It does not require energy. Size of the pores is the major limitation. Therefore, water and drugs with small molecular size are transported through this mechanism. Filtration mainly takes place in glomerulus.

CARRIER MEDIATED TRANSPORT

It is a rapid mode of transport. It demands a carrier, a substance in cell membrane that combines with a drug and takes that drug across the membrane. Such substances are called as ionophores. Specific ionophores are present for specific drugs. Active transport is carrier mediated transport that is against concentration gradient and it requires energy. If this carrier mediated transport is according to concentration gradient, it is called as facilitated diffusion. It does not demand energy.

Passive diffusion, filtration and facilitated transport do not need energy but carrier mediated active transport requires cellular energy.

PINOCYTOSIS

In this mode of transport individual cells take up particular molecules and bring them inside the cell. Utility of pinocytosis is controversial.

ABSORPTION

It is a transfer of drugs from the site of administration into circulation. In case of oral administration absorption refers to transfer of a drug from stomach/intestines into the blood while in case of intramuscular injection it refers to that from muscles into blood. Concept of absorption does not hold true from intravenous route of administration because drug is directly injected into blood. Bioavailability is a term that reflects absorption of drugs.

Absorption: Transfer of a drug from site of administration into circulation.

BIOAVAILABILITY

All drug that is administered may not go into the circulation (except for intravenous route). Some fraction is wasted at the site and some enters into the circulation. Bioavailability is the fraction of total administered drug that enters into circulation. It is the parameter that measures the rate and extent of absorption. Bioavailability of drugs is altered by various factors..

Bioavailability measures rate and extent of absorption of a drug.

Factors affecting absorption or bioavailability

Nature of drug
- Molecular weight
- Lipid solubility

Pharmaceutical factors
- Particle size
- Additives
- Formulation techniques

Host factors
- Genetic factors
- Disease status

Administration related factors
- Route
- Concentration
- pH at the site

Only for oral routes
- Disintegration
- Dissolution
- Enterohepatic circulation
- Food interactions
- Drug interactions
- First pass effect

1) Nature of the drug

Drugs with smaller molecular size are easily transported. Similarly lipid soluble drugs are absorbed fast. (Refer page 9)

2) Pharmaceutical factors

a) Small particle size improves absorption. Ultra micronized formulations of some drugs like griseofulvin are manufactured to improve the absorption of drugs.

b) Pharmaceutical adjuvants or excipients can alter bioavailability of drugs.

c) Pharmaceutical techniques like making sustained release tablets or enteric coated formulations alter the rate and extent of absorption.

3) Administration factors

a) Route of administration: Some drugs like penicillin G or insulin, if given orally, are destroyed in GI tract and bioavailability is zero. These agents are well absorbed by injectable routes. Bioavailability with intravenous route is 100%. For all other routes it is comparatively less.

b) Concentration of the medication: Diffusion of drug takes place according to the concentration gradient. Therefore if drug is administered in higher concentration absorption is faster.

c) pH at the site of administration: Acidic drugs are better absorbed in acidic medium and basic drugs in basic medium. The nature of drug and pH at the site decides the rate of absorption. (Refer page 9)

Intravenous route has 100% bioavailability.

4) Host factors

a) Disease status: any pathological change in absorbing area can alter absorption. Ex. Diarrhea increases motility of intestines and reduces absorption, in case of vascular collapse subcutaneously administered drug is not properly absorbed.

b) Genetic factors: (Refer page 46).

Diseases can alter bioavailability of drugs.

Specific factors related to oral route

a) Disintegration and dissolution: Disintegration time reflects time required for breaking of solid oral dosage form into granules. Dissolution rate refers to time required for drug to go into solution. Both these factors affect rate of absorption.

b) Drug-Food interaction or Drug-Drug interaction: If drug is taken orally along with food or some other drugs, their interaction in GI tract results in changes in rate and extent of absorption. (Refer page 40).

c) Enterohepatic circulation: Enterohepatic circulation refers to a circulation of an orally administered drug from intestine to liver and from liver to intestines.

Mechanism of enterohepatic circulation

Orally administered drug

↓

Drug in intestine

↓

Absorbed in portal circulation

↓

Goes to liver

↓

Drug is conjugated to glucuronic acid in liver

↓

Some part of conjugated drug is secreted along with bile into intestines

↓

Hydrolysis of conjugated drug into glucuronic acid and free drug in intestines

↓

Free drug again goes to liver and some part of that again comes to intestines. The process may be repeated for up to 8 times a day.

Ex. Drugs like sulindac, estradiol undergo this enterohepatic circulation.

Clinical implications of enterohepatic circulation

1) Enterohepatic circulation alters bioavailability.

2) The recycling of drug helps in prolonging the actions of some drugs.

d) First pass effect (Refer Page 21).

All these factors alter bioavailability of different drugs in different magnitude.

Enterohepatic circulation may prolong effects of drugs.

<u>Bioavailability: Clinical significance</u>

Figure 1.2 Represents absorption pattern of a drug

Figure 1.2 Absorption pattern of a drug and time-concentration curve

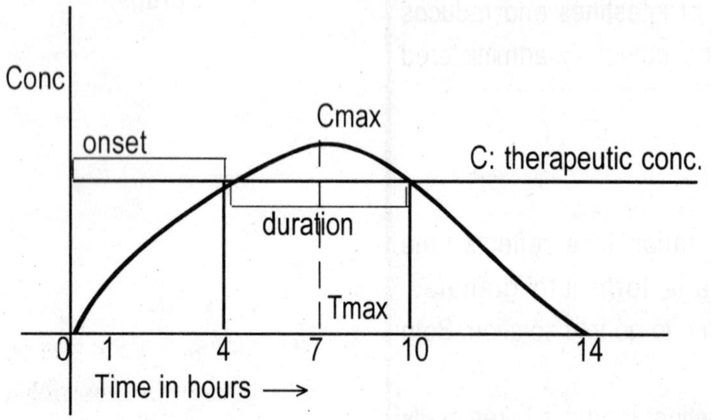

The figures on X-axis represent time and that on Y-axis concentration of drug in blood. At point 0 drug is administered. Concentration of drug in the blood gradually increases up to 7 hours. Then it starts declining and finally after 14 hours there is no drug in the blood.

The whole area under this curve (AUC) represents amount of drug absorbed. If similar type of graph is plotted after intravenous administration of drug, the bioavailability of that drug by oral route (F) is

Therapeutic concentration is one of the factors that decides onset and duration of action.

$$F = \frac{\text{AUC after oral administration}}{\text{AUC after intravenous administration}}$$

Line C in the graph represents therapeutic concentration. It means blood concentration of drug when is above that concentration then only that drug will have action. Four hours after taking the drug that concentration is achieved. Hence, 4 hours is the time required for the onset of action. Then up to 10 hours the concentration is above the therapeutic concentration and the action is continued. After that it goes down below therapeutic concentration and the action gets terminated. The period from 4 hours to 10 hours is duration of action. At 7 hours the concentration of drug in the body is maximum and it is termed as Cmax and the time 7 hours is termed as Tmax (time required to achieve maximum concentration). This graphical representation is termed as Time-concentration curve. Figure 1.3 represents Time-Concentration curves of three different drugs, from which there onset and duration can be compared.

Figure 1.3 Time concentration curves of three different drugs

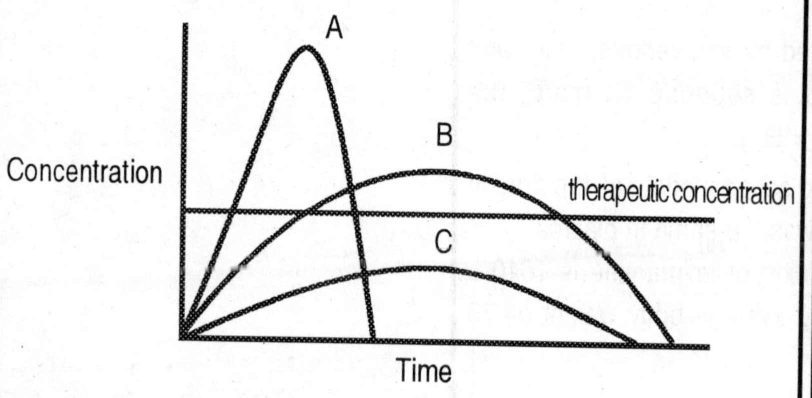

Drug A: Early onset - Short duration
Drug B: Late onset - Long duration
Drug C: Not effective therapeutically

Clinical significance of knowing bioavailability:

1) To decide the route of administration: If bioavailability of some drugs by specific route is zero or very less that route must be avoided.
Ex. Insulin is not given by oral route

Route of administration and dose is governed by bioavailability.

2) To decide the dose of a drug: Considering the fraction that is getting absorbed the administered dose must be appropriated.

3) Onset and duration of action of drugs can be predicted by knowing bioavailability pattern.

4) Bioequivalence: Bioequivalence is one of the major quality control criteria of the medications. Similar product units from all batches are supposed to release same amount of drug at same speed in the blood. In other words, bioequivalence must be proved. (The term bioequivalence concerns with rate and extent of absorption of drug in blood. It must be distinguished from therapeutic equivalence which relates to equal therapeutic effect with another product). When a new product is to be marketed, it must match bioequivalence to the present standard product.

DRUG DISTRIBUTION

Volume of distribution (Vd)

After absorption of a drug, a fraction gets attached to plasma proteins, and fraction remains free. The free portion is available for distribution all over the body. It is transferred into different compartments like extracellular fluids or inside the cells of different organs. The term 'volume of distribution' illustrates this distributed fraction of a drug.

Volume of distribution reflects distributed fraction of drug.

This term does not indicate real volume. It has no physiological significance and it is termed as apparent volume of distribution.

$$Vd = \frac{\text{Dose administered IV}}{\text{Plasma concentration}}$$

Ex. Suppose 500 mg drug is administered by intravenous route, and plasma concentration produced by it is suppose 10 mg/L, the apparent volume of distribution is 500/10 = 50 L

The volume reflects the volume that would accommodate all the drug in the body if the concentration throughout was the same in plasma

Ex. Average apparent volume of distribution of Imipramine is 1610 L and that of digoxin is 800 L. (considering average body weight as 70 kg).

Factors affecting distribution of drugs

Protein binding reduces distribution of drugs.

1) Drugs that have high protein binding, remain in vascular compartment (in blood) and are not distributed. Hence volume of distribution is less.

2) Drugs with poor lipid solubility do not penetrate into cells and remain in the extracellular compartment. They have less volume of distribution. Inversely lipid soluble drugs are widely distributed.

3) Specific transport mechanisms: Some drugs are specifically attached to some enzymes in the cell membrane. Ex. Digitalis to Na^+-K^+-ATPase or omeprazole to H^+-K^+-ATPase. This distribution regulates their action. Some drugs like tetracycline are remarkably distributed in bones and teeth and produce adverse effects at those sites.

4) Some disorders affect drug distribution. Ex. Obesity affects distribution of anesthetic agents that are highly fat soluble.

Drug redistribution:

During the process of distribution of drug, initially drug is mainly distributed to the organs which have high blood flow (brain, heart) and then to the organs with lesser blood flow (muscles, fats). Due to this distribution of drug, concentration of drug in the blood is reduced. To balance that, the drug from highly distributed areas comes back in the blood. This is redistribution of drug. It may be responsible for termination of action. But after repeated administrations when organs with lesser blood supply store sufficient amount of the drug, drug from these compartments, afterwards is transferred to blood and then to the compartment with more blood flow and the action is prolonged. The process of drug redistribution takes place when lipid solubility of drug is high. The concept of redistribution can be easily explained with the example of pentothal sodium induced anesthesia. Refer figure 1.4.

Drug redistribution prolongs duration of action of drug.

Figure 1.4 Redistribution of pentothal sodium

IV administration of pentothal sodium

Drug in blood

Rapid transport → Organs with more blood flow: brain → Anesthesia

Slow transport → Organs with lesser blood flow: fats

↓

Drop in plasma concentration.

↓

Pulling of drug from brain

↓

Termination of anesthesia

↓

Release of drug from fats into blood and then to brain

↓

Prolongation of action

Plasma protein binding

After absorption of a drug into blood, a fraction of drug is attached to some specific proteins in plasma and a fraction remains free. The attachment of drugs to plasma proteins is called as protein binding.

Plasma proteins:

Albumin and α acid glycoproteins are the two major plasma proteins involved in the process of protein binding. Acidic drugs are mainly attached to albumin while basic to α glycoprotein. Extent of protein binding varies according to the chemical nature of the drug. e.g. 90% of the absorbed fraction of doxycycline is bound to plasma proteins and only 10 % of gentamicin is bound to proteins. Warfarin, phenylbutazone, frusemide, diazepam are some drugs that are highly protein bound while ethosuccimide, amoxycillin, etc. are drugs with less protein binding.

Clinical significance of protein binding

1) The fraction of drug that is protein bound is pharmacologically inactive and only free drug can produce actions.

2) Protein bound drug and free drug are in equilibrium. When free drug after producing action is eliminated, protein bound fraction gets converted into free form and is made available for action. In a way, plasma proteins act as reservoirs and are responsible for prolonging the duration of action of drug.

Protein bound fraction of drugs is inert and serves as drug reservoir.

3) As long as drug is protein bound, it is not made available for the distribution all over the body, hence volume of distribution is inversely proportional to protein binding.

4) In disorders like renal or hepatic failure, plasma protein production is reduced. Subsequently protein bound fraction of drugs is also reduced and more drug is made available for the action and effect is exaggerated (compared to effect in normal individuals). Ex. In liver failure 71% of theophylline remains free compared to 35% in normal individuals. Proper adjustment of doses is required in these situations. Exactly opposite situation occurs in hyperproteinemia where protein bound fraction is increased and effects of drugs are reduced.

5) Drug interactions at protein binding sites:

If two drugs that share same plasma proteins are administered together, the one which has more affinity for the proteins displaces the second. Due to which, the free fraction of second drug increases and action is exaggerated. (Refer page 41).

Drugs can interact at protein binding sites.

Drug reservoirs

As the name suggests these drug reservoirs are the sites in the body that are capable of storing drugs. Plasma proteins and tissues like fat or muscles serve as drug resevoirs. Both are discussed earlier.

Clinical significance of drug reservoirs

When free drug in the body starts getting eliminated, drug from reservoirs, to maintain the equilibrium, is gradually released and the action is prolonged. High distribution of drug in certain organs is responsible for some adverse effects of drugs. Ex. Chloroquine by getting stored in retina produces ocular toxicity.

Accumulation of drug at specific site can result in local toxicity.

Distribution of drugs in specific compartments:

There are some specific compartments in the body that are characterized by barriers and they restrict entry of some drugs.

i) Blood brain and Blood CSF barrier,

ii) Placental barrier.

Blood Brain Barrier (BBB)

Nature has offered special protection to brain from drugs. Passage of drug in the brain is different from all organs. This is facilitated by different structure of capillaries in the CNS. Compared to normal blood vessels capillaries in CNS are differentiated in following ways:

a) They have tight junctions and no intracellular pores.

b) They do not contain pinocytes.

c) Additionally there is a covering of glial cells over the capillaries which also does not have pores.

These three differences in anatomical structure restrict the entry of drugs into brain. The drugs which are not lipid soluble or poorly lipid soluble can pass neither through capillary endothelium nor through the covering of glial cells (as both have no pores). Hence, brain allows only lipid soluble drugs to enter inside. Additionally in choroid plexus, similar type of barrier is present: Blood:CSF (Cerebrospinal fluid) barrier. It limits the passage of drug into CSF.

Clinical significance of blood brain barrier

1) The barrier protects brain from the toxic effects of lipid non soluble drugs and poisons.

2) During inflammation of meninges, permeability of BBB for drugs like penicillins or aminoglycosides is increased and they are effective.

3) Choice of drug in CNS disorders is largely governed by blood brain barrier Ex. Parkinsonism is a disease characterized by dopamine deficiency in brain. Dopamine, if administered externally, does not penetrate BBB. It is given in the precursor form i.e. L-dopa, which enters into brain and in brain it gets converted into dopamine.

4) BBB in fetus or neonates is not properly developed. So drugs that are to be used during pregnancy or delivery or in neonates must be selected accordingly.

Lipid soluble drugs penetrate BBB.

Inflammation of meninges improves permeability of BBB for drugs.

Placental barrier

Another barrier in the body is placental barrier, the role of which is controversial. Similar to BBB it also allows lipid soluble drugs but it is a weak barrier and almost all drugs can ultimately cross this barrier. Permeability of drugs through this barrier increases as pregnancy advances. Clinical significance of this barrier is discussed later in the section in teratogenicity (Refer Page 17).

Almost all drugs cross placental barrier.

BIOTRANSFORMATION OR METABOLISM OF DRUGS

Even though drugs are administered for the benefit of the body, body takes them as foreign bodies and tries to get rid of them. Biotransformation or metabolism of a drug is a process by which drug gets converted into a form that can be easily eliminated out of body. In other words, it is the conversion of drug into water soluble form. Ex. If some drug is getting excreted through urine and is lipid soluble, it will be reabsorbed from the cell membranes of tubular cell, but water soluble form will not get reabsorbed and is eliminated with urine.

Metabolism: conversion of a drug into excretable form.

The process of metabolism includes various chemical reactions. During these reaction original drug gets converted into metabolite or different metabolites.

After metabolism, drugs are converted into inactive or active metabolites.

Depending on the biological activity of metabolites, metabolism may be classified in following ways. -

I) Inactivation: It is the conversion of active drug into inactive metabolites. Most of the drugs are inactivated during the process of metabolism

II) Activation:

A) In this situation the metabolite is biologically active. Ex. Diazepam is a drug, which after metabolism gets converted into oxazepam which also is biologically active. The drug that is administered and the metabolite produced, both are active.

B) In some situations, a pharmacologically inactive substance, after metabolism, gets converted into a pharmacologically active substance. The drug administered is inactive and metabolite is active. Ex. L.dopa is pharmacologically inactive. After metabolism, it gets converted into active metabolite dopamine. Such drugs are called as prodrugs.

Metabolism activates prodrugs

Table 1.2 Prodrugs

Prodrug	Active metabolites
Bacampicillin	Ampicillin
Benorylate	Aspirin + Paracetamol
Enalapril	Enalaprilat
L-Dopa	Dopamine

Prodrugs can improve absorption, distribution and reduce toxicity of drugs.

Clinical significance of prodrugs:

1) Prodrugs, sometimes are better absorbed than drugs. Ex. Talampicillin, a prodrug of ampicillin is absorbed better than ampicillin.

2) Prodrugs can reduce toxicity: Benorylate produces less GI adverse effects than aspirin.

3) Administration of prodrugs can help in proper distribution of drugs. Ex. L.dopa (a prodrug of dopamine) can cross BBB. (Dopamine- the active form of drug cannot).

Figure 1.5 Consequences of metabolism

Active drug	→	Inactive metabolite
Active drug	→	Active metabolite
Inactive drug	→	Active metabolite

Metabolism mainly takes place in liver but kidney, intestines, lungs, skin, etc. are also capable of metabolizing various drugs.

Chemical reactions involved in the process of biotransformation:
The reactions are divided into two phases: phase I and phase II.

Table 1.3 Comparison of phase I and phase II reactions

PHASE I	PHASE II
1) Non-synthetic reactions	1) Synthetic reactions
2) Includes processes like oxidation, reduction etc.	2) Conjugation is the main chemical process
3) Metabolites of phase I reactions can be active, inactive or toxic	3) Metabolites of phase II reaction are necessarily inactive

Phase I reactions normally produce active metabolites while Phase II reactions produce inactive metabolites.

Drugs are eliminated from the body by 4 different alternatives.

1) Some drugs are eliminated unchanged without metabolism.

2) Some drugs undergo only phase I reactions and are eliminated.

3) Some drugs undergo only phase II reactions and are eliminated.

4) For some drugs phase I and II both reactions are required for their elimination.

Table 1.4 Chemical reactions involved in phase I

Reaction	Subtypes	Agents
Oxidation	Aromatic hydroxylation Aliphatic hydroxylation Sulfoxidation, Epoxidation etc.	Barbiturates Benzodiazepines
Reduction	AZO reduction, Nitro reduction Sulfide reduction	Disulfiram Chloramphenicol
Hydrolysis		Pethidine, INH

During Phase I reactions, highly reactive intermediates like epoxides or superoxides can be generated. These intermediates are responsible for various toxic effects of drugs. Antioxidant substances in the body reduce this toxicity. Externally administered antioxidant drugs have similar type of action.

Phase II reactions:

Metabolites generated from these reactions are necessarily inactive and water soluble. These reactions actually involve combination of drug (or metabolite from phase I reaction) to a water soluble molecule that results in water soluble conjugate. All reactions in phase II involve conjugation

Table 1.5 Chemical reactions involved in phase II

Reaction	Example
Glucuronide conjugation	Aspirin
Glutathione conjugation	Morphine
Glycine conjugation	Salicylates
Acetylation	INH, Sulfonamides
Methylation	Noradrenaline, Histamine

Phase I and phase II reactions take place sequentially or simultaneously.

Enzymes involved in the process of metabolism

Chemical reactions involved in metabolism (both phase I and II) require enzymes. For some drugs there are specific enzymes (e.g. alcohol dehydrogenase for alcohol). For majority of drugs these enzymes are not specific and different drugs can be metabolized by same enzymes. These enzymes are of two types.

1) Microsomal enzymes: These enzymes are situated on endoplasmic reticulum in liver (also in kidney, lungs), most common example is cytochrome P 450. They are required for oxidation, reduction, hydrolysis (from phase I) and glucuronic acid conjugation (from phase II) reactions.

Hepatic microsomal enzyme induction reduces duration and magnitude of action of drugs.

2) Non microsomal enzymes: These enzymes are located in cytoplasm and mitochondria (mainly of liver). Conjugases, esterases, amidases are some of the enzymes from this class. Non microsomal enzymes are mainly involved in hydrolysis (from phase I) and all phase II reactions except glucuronidation.

Enzyme induction

Administration of various substances in the body can increase the synthesis and activity of hepatic microsomal enzymes. This enzyme induction alters effects of drugs in following manner.

Drug administration (along with some enzyme inducers)
↓ ← Induced enzymes
Increase in metabolism of drug
↓
Increase in rate of elimination/inactivation
↓
Reduced duration of action of drug
Reduction in magnitude of action of drug

In this way enzyme induction results in reduction in duration and magnitude of action of drugs.

Substances capable of inducing microsomal enzymes:

A large number of substances can induce enzymes. Some of them are Barbiturates, DDT, Alcohol, Phenytoin, Tobacco, etc. These substances induce hepatic microsomal enzymes and alter effects of the drugs that are administered with them.

Clinical significance of enzyme induction

1) If drugs like oral contraceptives or anticoagulants are administered along with barbiturates (enzyme inducers), barbiturates can induce the enzymes that are required for metabolism of these agents and failure of activity of these agents is possible.

2) If a drug is to be administered along with some enzyme inducer, proper adjustment of dose is required.

3) Development of tolerance: Alcohol, after chronic consumption, induces enzyme that are involved in self (alcohol) metabolism. That is the reason why the effects of alcohol are reduced after chronic consumption.

Enzyme induction leads to tolerance.

4) Increase in the rate of metabolism sometimes is a reason for toxicity if metabolites are toxic. Ex. Metabolites of paracetamol are hepatotoxic or metabolites of Na nitroprusside can produce toxic psychosis.

5) Therapeutic scope : In liver failure where hepatic enzyme production is hampered, external administration of enzyme inducers can be beneficial. Induced metabolism can also be used therapeutically in case of poisoning to increase the rate of elimination of poisons by promoting metabolism.

Enzyme inhibition

This situation is exactly opposite to enzyme induction.

Drug administration (along with some enzyme inhibitors)

↓ ← Inhibited enzymes

Reduced metabolism of drug

↓

Reduced elimination/inactivation

↓

Increased duration and magnitude of action of drug

Increased accumulation and toxicity of drug

In this way enzyme inhibition results in exaggerated actions of drug.

Drugs that are capable of inhibiting metabolizing enzymes:
Dicoumarol, Ketoconazole, Cimetidine, Sulfonamides, etc.

Clinical implications of enzyme inhibition:
Dicoumarol, if administered along with phenytoin, inhibits enzymes that are involved in the metabolism of phenytoin and phenytoin toxicity is enhanced. Similarly, disulfiram and metronidazole, if given with alcohol, inhibit enzyme aldehyde dehydrogenase (enzyme that metabolizes alcohol) and causes acetaldehyde syndrome. Proper adjustments of dose of a drug is desirable if its metabolism is expected to be inhibited due to administration of another drug. Many drugs are known to produce their effects through enzyme inhibition.

Inhibition of hepatic microsomal enzyme increases toxicity of drugs.

First-pass Effect or presystemic elimination of drugs

In case of some drugs, a fraction of orally administered drug when is metabolized before going to systemic circulation, the phenomenon is called as first pass effect or presystemic elimination.

Mechanism of first pass effect:
Orally administered drug

↓

Drug in gastrointestinal tract -
Fraction 'x' of total drug is metabolized in GI tract

↓

Through portal circulation drug goes to liver

Fraction 'y' of absorbed drug is metabolized in liver and remaining fraction 'z' goes into circulation and is made available for action

Thus fraction 'x+y' is metabolized before going into the circulation and is not available for the biological action. Only fraction 'z' is available for the biological action. This is presystemic elimination of a drug.

Presystemic metabolism: Some orally administered drugs are metabolized before producing actions

Drugs that undergo presystemic elimination: Nitroglycerine, morphine propranolol, amitriptyline, etc.

Clinical implications of first pass effect
1) Deciding the route: Drugs with high first pass effect if given orally, a large fraction may not be available for the action. In other words their bioavailability by oral route is poor. Alternative route like sublingual route can be preferred in such situations. Ex. Sublingual nitroglycerine.

2) Dose adjustment: The fraction getting presystemically metabolized reduces the bioavailability of drug. Proper adjustment of doses must be done considering the metabolized fraction.

3) The decision of dose is further complicated by variation in the magnitude of presystemic elimination in individual patient.

4) In liver disorders presystemic elimination is inhibited due to pathology in the liver. When the expected presystemic metabolism does not take place, excess drug is made available in the systemic circulation and exaggerated action or toxicity is observed. Same problem is possible when two drugs having first pass effect are administered together.

Similar type of presystemic metabolism sometimes takes place in skin after transdermal administration of drugs.

Drugs with high first pass effect are usually not administered by oral route; or proper adjustment of dose is essential

Figure 1.6 Factors affecting metabolism of drugs
Genetic factors
Liver disorders
Enzyme induction and inhibition
Route of administration
Drug interactions

Liver disorders alter metabolism of drugs, therefore drugs are used with caution in liver disorders.

All these factors are discussed in section "Factors affecting actions of drugs". (Refer page 53).

ELIMINATION OR EXCRETION OF DRUGS

Elimination or excretion refers to the removal of drug out of the body. Drugs are eliminated without metabolism or after metabolism. Drugs are eliminated by different routes.

Drugs are eliminated through urine, stools, exhaled air, breast milk, tears, sweat, saliva.

Various routes of excretion:

Renal elimination: This is the most common route of elimination. Three processes in kidney govern the rate and amount of elimination.

Refer figure 1.7

Figure 1.7 Renal elimination of drugs

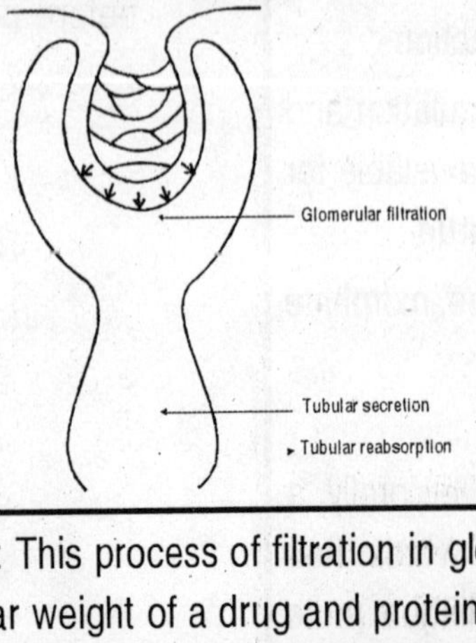

i) Glomerular filtration: This process of filtration in glomerulus is mainly controlled by molecular weight of a drug and protein binding of a drug. A drug with molecular weight less than 10,000 and which is not protein bound is easily filtered. G.F.R. (Glomerular Filtration Rate) is a parameter that measures the rate of this process. Since creatinine is cleared principally by filtration, measurement of rate of renal creatinine clearance is considered as standard guideline.

ii) Tubular secretion : This is an active transfer of a drug in proximal tubule. Charged molecules are usually transported by this route. Two different systems of transport are present for acidic transport (penicillin, uric acid etc.) and basic transport (amphetamine, cimetidine).

Rate of renal elimination of drug is governed by glomerular filtration, tubular secretion and tubular reabsorption

iii) Tubular reabsorption: When concentration of drug in renal tubules exceeds that in plasma, flow of drug is in opposite direction i.e. from tubules into renal blood vessels. During this passive reabsorption process tubular cell membranes act as lipid barrier and only lipid soluble fraction of drug is reabsorbed back in the blood.

Fecal elimination of drugs

Drugs are removed with feces in 4 different situations.

1) Unabsorbed part of the drug

2) Some drugs like neomycin are not intended to be absorbed and are supposed to act in intestines. After the action they are removed with stools.

3) Some drugs diffuse back from blood into intestines

4) Many drugs after going to liver are secreted into bile and eliminated along with it into stools. Ex. Neomycin, doxycycline.

Pulmonary elimination of drugs

Pulmonary elimination refers to removal of drugs through exhaled air. This is a major route of elimination of volatile anesthetics and alcohol.

Elimination of drugs in breast milk

The amount of drug that gets eliminated in breast milk usually is not significant for the mother but may be potentially toxic for the baby. As milk is slightly acidic in nature as compared to plasma, basic drugs are preferably concentrated in milk. Following are some of the drugs that can have adverse effects in babies if administered to lactating mothers.

Drug to mother	-	Effects on baby
Corticosteroids	-	Suppression of adrenal functions
Sulfonamides	-	Hemolytic anemia, kernicterus
Chloramphenicol	-	Gray baby syndrome/bone marrow depression

Elimination in breast milk limits use of drugs in lactating mothers.

These drugs are usually contraindicated in lactating mothers. Saliva, sweat, tears are some additional routes of elimination

Clinical implications of drug elimination

1) In old age or in case of renal disorders the altered renal function can be responsible for decreased elimination of drugs and adjustment of doses may be required.

2) Rate of urinary excretion of some drugs can be increased by altering pH of the urine for therapeutic applications.

Alterations in renal elimination of drug can be used therapeutically.

Ex. In case of barbiturate poisoning urine is made alkaline. Being acidic, barbiturates in urine remain in ionized form and are not reabsorbed and elimination is increased.

3) Some drugs act at the level of excretion. Ex. Probenecid inhibits tubular reabsorption of uric acid and promotes elimination. Hence the drug is called as uricosuric drug and is used in gout (a disease in which uric acid crystals are formed in joints).

4) Drug interactions at the level of excretion. Penicillin and probenecid when are given together, probenecid gets excreted at the place of penicillin and reduces excretion of penicillin. This prolongs the duration of action of penicillin.

5) Drugs that are eliminated in breast milk and can cause undesirable effects in babies are contraindicated in lactating mothers.
Ex. Sulfonamides, chloramphenicol.

6) Medicolegal aspects: Amount of alcohol in exhaled air is measured by breathanalysers and it has legal importance in accidents. Presence of arsenic in hair gives an idea about arsenic poisoning.

Elimination kinetics

Clearance reflects elimination of drugs

Clearance is a term or figure that reflects elimination of drugs from the body. Ex : If clearance of a drug is 20 ml/min, it means every 20 ml of plasma or blood is completely free of drug in one minute. In other words, clearance is a volume of plasma or blood that is free of drug per unit time. Clearance is denoted by CL and is calculated by following formula

$$CL = \frac{\text{Rate of elimination}}{\text{Plasma concentration}}$$

Ex. Suppose concentration of a drug in the blood is 3 mg/ml and rate of elimination is 60 mg/min. Then clearance = 60/3 = 20 ml/min. Clearance can also be expressed in terms of ml/min/kg.

Depending on the capacity of body to eliminate different drugs the pharmacokinetics is classified into two types ; first order kinetics and zero order kinetics.

First order kinetics or Exponential kinetics

In case of most of the drugs when concentration of drugs in body increases the amount eliminated also increases. When the rate of elimination of drug is directly proportional to concentration of drug, it is first order kinetics. If concentration of drug in body increases, the elimination also increases. In other words, a *fraction* of total drug that is getting eliminated is constant. Most of the drugs fortunately follow first order kinetics and hence their elimination in the body is exponential and predictable. Refer figure 1.8

Zero order kinetics

In case of some drugs, capacity of body to metabolize the drugs is limited. Therefore even if concentration of these drugs in blood is increased, elimination does not increase in the same proportion. In other words, it is not the fraction of total drug that gets eliminated but it is the *fixed amount* of drug that gets eliminated remains constant. (Refer figure 1.8). This type of kinetics is termed **as saturation kinetics** because capacity of body to metabolize the drug gets saturated. Zero order kinetics leads to reduced elimination and increased accumulation of drugs. Ex. Drugs like alcohol, phenytoin follow first order kinetics initially and then switch on to zero order kinetics. This leads to accumulation and exaggerated actions of these drugs. That is why effect of alcohol increases improportionately after excessive consumption. Zero order kinetics alters half-life of a drug in unpredictable manner

Drugs that follow zero order kinetics are accumulated in body.

Figure 1.8 First and zero order kinetics

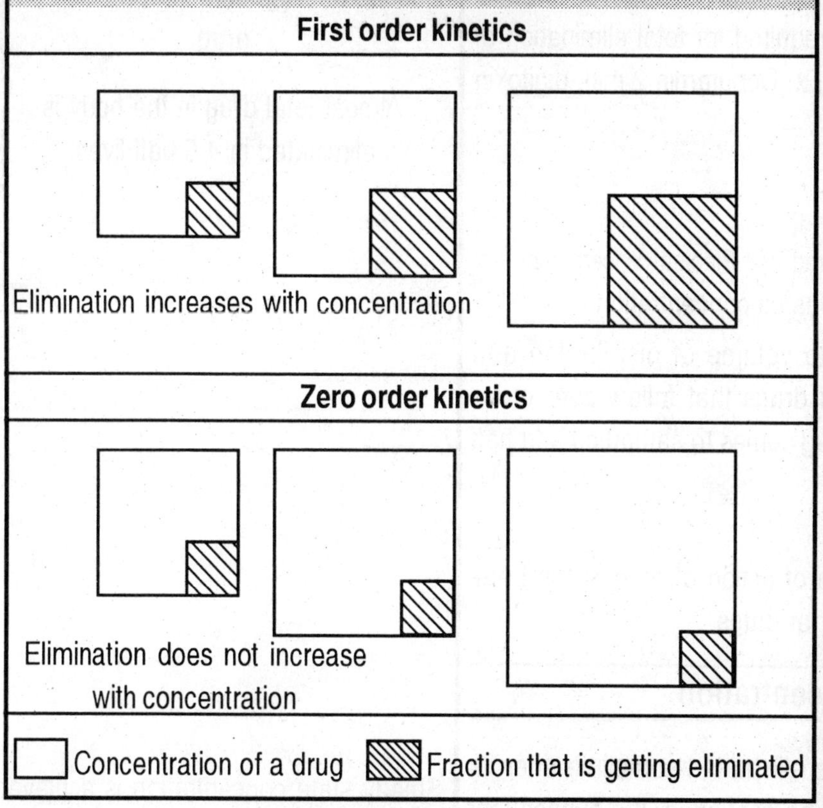

First order kinetics: Fixed fraction gets eliminated

Zero order kinetics: Fixed quantity gets eliminated.

Elimination half-Life ($t_{1/2}$)

Elimination half-life of a drug is the time taken for its plasma concentration to reduce to half of its original amount.

Suppose a drug is administered by IV route at 0 hours. At that point all the drug is in blood and drug concentration is maximum. Then there is sudden fall in drug concentration due to distribution of drug in various compartments. Then there is a further gradual fall due to elimination of drug. Gradually all the drug is removed out of the body. Suppose, immediately after administration (0 hours) plasma concentration is

40 μg/ml. Gradually the concentration gets reduced and say after 4 hours the concentration becomes 20 μg/ml (half of its original amount). Four hours is half life of the drug. In next 4 hours, half of that gets eliminated and the concentration becomes 10 μg/ml and in next 4 hours concentration will be 5 μg/ml and so on. If it is converted into percentage form, the picture is as follows. Refer figure 1.9.

Half of the drug in the body is eliminated in 1 half-life.

Figure 1.9 Half-lives of drug

Time	%. elimination	% fraction in the blood
0 hrs	0 %	100 %
after 4 hrs.	50 %	50 %
after 8 hrs.	50 + 25 = 75 %	25 %
after 4+4+4 = 12 hrs.	50+25+12.5 = 87.5 %	12.5 %
after 4+4+4+4 = 16 hrs.	50+25+12.5+6.25 = 93.15 %	6.25 %

Thus, after around 4 half lives, a major fraction of drug is eliminated and only negligible fraction remains in blood (unless another dose is administered) so total 4-5 half lives are required for total elimination of drugs. Half life varies from drug to drug. Ex. Dobutamin 2 min, digitoxin 7 days, diazepam 40 hours, etc.

Halt life decides duration of action of a drug.

Almost total drug in the body is eliminated in 4-5 half lives.

Measurement of half-life ($t_{1/2}$)

$t_{1/2} = 0.693 \times V/CL$

V = volume of distribution = Dose administered IV / Plasma concentration

CL = Clearance = Rate of eliminations/ Plasma concentration

Thus half life is directly proportional to volume of distribution and inversely to the elimination. In case of drugs that follow zero order kinetics, capacity of body to eliminate drug comes to saturation and half life does not remain constant.

Clinical significance of half life

Half life gives basic idea about duration of action of drug in the body and helps in deciding dosing frequency of drugs

Steady state concentration

Depending on the half life, all drug gets eliminated sometime after its administration. If activity of a drug is to be continued, the subsequent doses must be administered with the objective of maintaining steady state concentration above therapeutic concentration. This steady state is the state in which rate of elimination of drug is equal to rate of administration and amount of drug in the body is fairly constant: plateau concentration. In case of IV administration this is achieved by continuous infusion. The same concentration is achieved with intermittent oral or IV doses but only difference is that there are peaks and troughs, but the mean concentration remains fairly constant. If drug is given at constant rate (continuous or intermittent) it is after 5 half lives, steady state concentration is usually achieved. Steady state

Steady state concentration is achieved by matching rates of administration and elimination.

concentration can be calculated by following formula -
Steady state concentration = dose rate/clearance

Loading dose and maintenance dose

After administration, when drug levels in the body reach above therapeutic concentration, the action is initiated and it is maintained till the concentration remains above that concentration. Refer figure 1.10.

Figure 1.10 Loading and maintenance dose

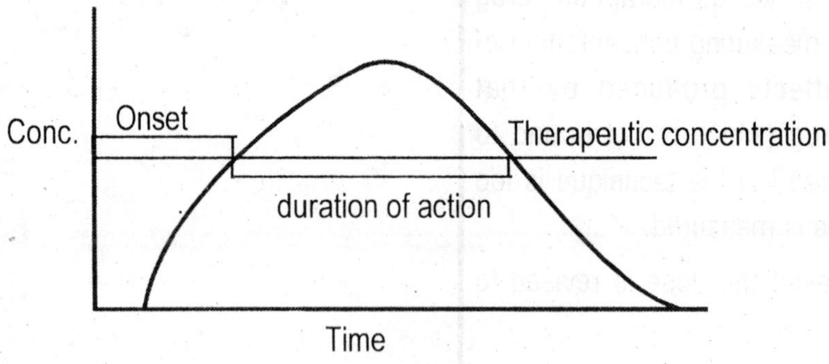

Loading dose achieves therapeutic concentration and maintenance dose keeps it above that concentration.

Loading dose: It is a high initial dose (or multiple doses) administered at the initiation of therapy to achieve therapeutic concentration. It is measured as -

$$\text{Loading dose} = \frac{\text{Target conc} \times V}{F}$$

V = Volume of distribution F = Bioavailability

Maintenance dose: These are multiple doses administered after loading dose to maintain the level of drug above therapeutic concentration and below toxic concentration.

$$\text{Maintenance dose} = \frac{\text{Target conc} \times CL}{F}$$

CL = Clearance F = Bioavailability

Ex. Atropinisation (high initial doses of atropine) in organophosphorus poisoning, or initial high dose of chloroquine in malaria are the common examples of loading doses. Subsequent doses are required in less quantities to maintain the effective concentration.

Therapeutic drug monitoring (TDM)

Administration of a specific dose produces a specific concentration of drug in the circulation that results in certain action.

Specific dose of a drug
↓
Specific plasma concentration
↓
Specific effect of drug

There are three different correlations between these three parameters.

i) Correlation between dose and concentration

ii) Correlation between concentration and effect

iii) Correlation between dose and effect

Usually depending on therapeutic calculation and for the sake of convenience the correlation between dose and effect is used to monitor a patient. But there is a vast interpersonal variation in this correlation, which is not acceptable in certain crucial situations. Correlation between plasma concentration and effect is comparatively much reliable and can be used for monitoring patients. This is termed as therapeutic drug monitoring. In simple words TDM means measuring concentration of drugs in blood and checking the effects produced by that concentration. Ideally free fraction of drug (which is not bound to proteins) in the plasma should be measured but the technique is too difficult and usually total drug in the plasma is measured.

Correlation between plasma concentration and effects of drug is highly reliable.

If the expected level of drug is not achieved the dose is revised to attain the expected level.

$$\text{New dose rate} = \frac{\text{Previous dose rate x Expected concentration}}{\text{Actual concentration}}$$

Situations where TDM is crucial or possible:

i) In case of drugs which are known for high interpersonal variations Ex. Lithium

ii) Drugs with narrow therapeutic range. If slight increase in concentration produces toxicity and slight reduction takes away the activity, TDM becomes desirable. Ex. Digoxin. Therapeutic effect of digoxin is not achieved below 0.8 ng/ml and toxic effects are observed after 3 ng/ml.

iii) TDM, especially is useful when effects of drugs can not easily be judged. Ex. Effects of antipsychotic drugs on mood.

iv) During therapeutic failure of some drugs TDM helps in checking patient compliance (to confirm whether patient is really taking a drug or not).

Situation where TDM is not required or is impossible

TDM sometimes not required, sometimes not possible.

i) In case of drugs where effect can easily be measured, TDM is not required. Ex. Antihypertensive effect of drugs can be measured by checking BP rather than TDM.

ii) Actions of some drugs do not depend on concentration. The action is 'hit and run' type. Once action is started, it is independent of concentration. Ex. Antiplatelet action of aspirin. In such a situation TDM has no role.

Prolonging actions of drugs

Duration of action of drug is a major factor that decides the frequency of administration of a drug and frequency of administration decides compliance. Increased frequency grossly reduces patient compliance. Techniques that prolong the duration of action reduce frequency of administration and improve patient compliance. Some dosage schedules demand interruption in sleep, which can be avoided by prolonging duration of action. Different techniques (at different levels) are used to prolong the duration of action

Duration of action of drug can be prolonged at various levels; formulation, administration, absorption, distribution, metabolism, excretion.

Long acting agents improve patient compliance

Table 1.6 Techniques used to prolong duration of action

Level	Alteration or technique	Examples
Drug chemical	Synthesizing new derivatives by altering chemical structure	Long acting derivatives of benzodiazepines
Formulation	Extended release preparations or depot preparations	Insulin preparations, steroid depots
Administration	High dose administration (may not be practicable always)	
Absorption	Combining the drug molecule with some other molecules that delays absorption.	Lente insulin, procaine penicillin
Distribution	Adrenaline, when given along with local anesthetics, produces vasoconstriction at the site and reduces distribution of drugs keeping maximum drug at the site of administration	Lignocaine with adrenaline
Protein binding	Increase in protein binding results in reduction in immediate distribution of drug which subsequently prolongs the duration of action.	long acting sulfonamides have more protein binding
Metabolism	If two drugs are given together and one drug inhibits the metabolism of the second, the duration of action of second drug is prolonged	Carbidopa inhibits enzyme decarboxylase which is required for metabolism of L-dopa
Excretion	One drug can reduce elimination of another drug	Probenecid reduces renal elimination of penicillin.

PHARMACODYNAMICS

Pharmacodynamics reflects what a drug does to a body. It includes details of desired and undesired effects. Drugs can produce effects in a variety of ways.

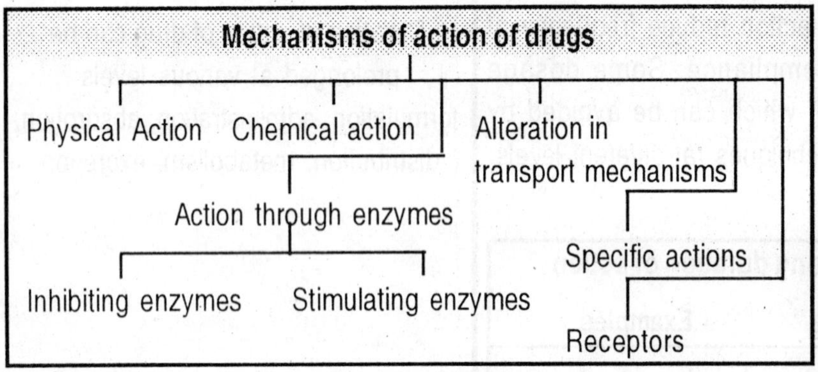

1) Physical action: Ex. Bulk laxatives absorb water and swell. They form a mass in large intestine and facilitate the passage of stools. This mechanism involves a physical action.

2) Chemical action: Antacids neutralize acid in the stomach and reduce acidity. It is due to the chemical reaction of neutralization.

3) Action through enzymes: This is one of the common modes of action. Enzymes are substances (proteins), which do not take part in the chemical reactions but they have potential to stimulate reactions. Some drugs, due to their action on enzymes, alter reactions in the body. Most of the therapeutic applications of these drugs involve inhibition of enzyme controlled reactions.

a) Competitive action

Ex. Angiotensin I gets converted in the body into Angiotensin II, which produces vasoconstriction. Angiotensin converting enzyme (ACE) is required for this conversion. Lisinopril is a drug (ACE inhibitor) that is structurally similar to Angiotensin I. After administration of lisinopril the enzyme ACE gets attached to lisinopril. It reduces availability of ACE for the conversion of Angiotensin I to II. In the same way sulfonamides compete with enzyme PABA for enzyme folate synthetase.

b) Noncompetitive enzymatic action

Prostaglandins are the substances that are required for process of inflammation. Cycloxygenase is the enzyme that is responsible for production of prostaglandins. NSAIDs (ibuprofen, diclofenac, etc.) inhibit this enzyme and prevent formation of prostaglandins and reduce inflammation. Similarly omeprazole inhibits enzyme H^+ K^+ ATPase and prevents formation of acid in stomach.

c) Action by stimulating enzymes

Drugs like streptokinase or urokinase stimulate enzyme plasminogen and promote breakdown of blood clot. Pralidoxime activates enzyme cholinesterase and is used in OP poisoning.

4) Alteration in transport systems

Drugs can alter entry and exit of different ions inside cell. Ex. Calcium channel blockers like nifedipine, verapamil prevent entry of calcium inside cell and prevent contraction of muscles. Vasodilators like hydralazine open K^+ channels and promote entry of K^+ inside the cells and produce relaxation of vascular smooth muscles.

5) Specific actions

i) Drugs can alter constitution of cell membrane. Ex. General anesthetics alter lipids, protein and water in the nerve cell membrane and produce anesthetic action.

ii) Drugs can alter specific metabolic processes inside the human cell and affect microorganisms. Ex. Penicillins inhibit cell wall synthesis of microorganisms but not that of human cells. In case of drugs like 5 fluorouracil - (anticancer drug) the drug gets incorporated in RNA and produces the action.

Receptors

Majority of drugs act through receptors.

Most of the currently used drugs produce their action through receptors. Receptor is a macromolecule situated on the surface of cell or inside the cell that recognizes and binds with specific molecules producing specific effects in cells. In brief, it is the site that provides space for attachment of some specific substances and regulates the functioning of cell.

Receptors provide site for natural substances and for drugs.

Physiological receptors

These receptors provide site for physiological substances in human body. Ex. Adrenergic receptors provide space for adrenaline.

Drug receptors

These receptors specifically provide space for attachment of specific drugs. Ex. Benzodiazepines get attached to benzodiazepine receptors.

Affinity

It is the capacity of a substance to get attached to the receptor. Ex. Adrenaline has affinity for adrenergic receptors.

Intrinsic activity

It is the capacity of a substance to bring out some changes (or produce some action) after getting attached to receptor. Ex. Adrenaline after getting attached to adrenergic receptors generates cyclic AMP and increases force of contraction and rate of heart. Action of a drug and effects of a drug are two different things. Action means the changes in receptor due to combination of a drug with receptor and drug effect means biological effects that can be observed after administration of a drug.

Agonist

It is a substance that gets attached to a receptor and produces some conformational changes in receptor (or produce some action). In a way, it has got affinity and intrinsic activity. Ex. Adrenaline gets attached to adrenergic receptors and produces increase in heart rate, so it is agonist of adrenergic receptors. Drugs which are structurally similar to adrenaline have the same action and are called adrenergic agonists. Ex. Terbutaline is adrenergic agonist. Natural neurotransmitters like adrenaline get destroyed in body immediately. Compared to that artificially administered agonists have longer duration of action. If agonist has selectivity for particular receptor, quality of effect is superior. Nonselectivity leads to stimulation of large number of receptors and widespread undesired effects.

Competitive antagonist

A substance that gets attached to receptor but doesn't produce any action is called as an antagonist. Antagonist has got affinity for that receptor but no intrinsic activity. Antagonists usually are structurally similar to agonists. Ex. Propranolol is a drug that gets attached to beta adrenegic receptors on the heart and prevents attachment of adrenaline (which naturally is present in the body) to the receptors. This prevents increase in heart rate or reduces heart rate. Antagonists are termed as blockers of receptors.

Agonist has got affinity and intrinsic activity. Antagonist has got affinity but no intrinsic activity.

Partial agonist

This substance has both affinity and intrinsic activity but intrinsic activity is less than agonist. They partially block the receptors and partially stimulate receptors. Ex. Pindolol is actually a blocker but it also can partially stimulate some receptors. So it is called as partial agonist of beta receptors.

Inverse agonist

It is a substance that gets attached to receptors, produces action but the action is exactly opposite to that of agonist (They must be differentiated from antagonists which do not produce any action) Ex. Beta carbolines are inverse agonists of benzodiazepine receptors and produce actions that are exactly opposite to benzodiazepines.

Inverse agonist produces actions opposite to agonist.

Figure 1.11 Drugs and receptors

Drug	Affinity	Activity
Antagonist	✔	No
Agonist	✔	Full
Partial agonist	✔	Less
Inverse agonist	✔	Opposite

Spare receptors

Ex. Suppose a drug, after getting attached to receptors on the heart, produces increase in heart rate. Maximum increase in the heart rate that can be produced by that drug is say by 20. This action can be provided by occupying only 5% of the receptors. Remaining 95% receptors even if are blocked, the same rise in heart rate is achieved. The remaining receptors work as spare receptors.

Silent receptors

Some receptors even after their attachment to agonists are not activated. They do not have capacity to produce positive action and are termed as silent receptors. If active receptors are blocked for a long time, the silent receptors can be converted into active receptors.

Selectivity of drugs for receptor improves the quality of action. Non-selectivity increases chances of undesired effects.

Regulation of receptors

Receptor down-regulation: When receptors are exposed to agonists for a long time, the number of receptors and their sensitivity for the agonist are reduced. This is receptor down-regulation. Some times receptors that are situated on the surface are internalized (taken inside the cell) and number of available receptors for attachment of drug is reduced. When the agonist is discontinued, the activity of receptors reappears. **Clinical significance:** Salbutamol is an agonist of beta receptors. When it is given in bronchial asthma it stimulates β receptors on lungs and dilates bronchi. If given for prolonged period, β receptors loose their sensitivity for salbutamol and effect is gradually reduced. To avoid this, some drug free period must be given by changing the drug. Tachyphylaxis is the similar type of reduction in effect which is observed after repeated administration of drugs.

Prolonged exposure to agonist reduces effects of agonists.

Receptor up-regulation: If receptors are blocked for a long time, the number and sensitivity of the receptors for agonist are increased. This is called as receptor up-regulation. It is also reversible. **Clinical significance:** Propranolol is an antagonist or blocker of β receptors on the heart. If propranolol is administered for a long period, number of beta receptors on the heart is increased. When administration of propranolol is suddenly stopped, the large number of receptors are exposed to natural agonist adrenaline and there is exaggerated increase in heart rate. This is an effect which is exactly opposite to propranolol. It is withdrawal effect.

Sudden withdrawal of antagonist produces withdrawal reactions.

Mechanisms of receptor actions

Receptors regulate functions of cells by different mechanisms. According to mechanism they are classified in different types:

I) Receptors with intrinsic ion channels

These receptors are on the surface of cell and contain ion channels. Different receptors have channels for different ions like Na^+, K^+, Cl^-, etc. Stimulation of receptors by drugs alters flow of ions through these channels and cellular actions are regulated. E.g.. Nicotinic receptors or 5HT receptors.

II) Enzyme receptors

These receptors are actually enzymes (Ex. Tyrosine kinase). One part of the receptor is outside the cell while one is inside. Drug or agonist binds to the outer part and stimulates phosphorylation of receptors, which subsequently phosphorylates intracellular proteins and produces actions. Ex. Insulin receptors.

III) Gene associated receptors

These receptors are situated inside the cell and are associated with genes. Drug enters into cell and gets attached to these receptors. Stimulation of these receptors alters gene expression of the cell and produces different actions. Ex. Steroid receptors.

IV) G protein coupled receptors

G protein means GTP activated protein. G proteins are of different types. Some receptors are associated with these G proteins. Agonist stimulates receptors. The stimulated receptors produce action through G proteins in following three pathways:

1) Action through adenylyl cyclase and cAMP

Agonist

↓

Stimulation of receptors

↓

Activation of G proteins

↓

Activation of adenylyl cyclase

↓

Accumulation of cAMP

↓

Various actions

Ex Dopamine receptors, H_2 receptors

2) Action through IP_3/DAG

Agonist

↓

Stimulation of receptors

↓

Activation of G proteins

↓

Activation of phospholipase C

↓

Generation of IP_3 / DAG

(Inositol triphosphate/diacylglycerol)

↓

Increased intracellular calcium

↓

Various actions

Ex. Beta receptors, histamine receptors

3) **Action through G protein associated ion channels.**

Agonist

↓

Stimulation of receptors

↓

Activation of G proteins

↓

Alteration in the flow of ion channels

↓

Actions

Ex. β_2 receptors

Some G proteins are inhibitory proteins and produce actions opposite to that of stimulatory proteins.

Dose response curve. (DRC)

Biological effect of drug increases according to the increase in dose administered. This correlation is observed only up to a certain extent. After that even if the dose is increased, effect remains the same. If these observations are plotted in graphical form, the presentation is termed as Dose Response Curve of a drug for that effect. If doses are plotted on X axis and responses on Y, the shape of the graph is hyperbola. For the sake of calculation convenience, instead of dose, log dose is used on X axis, and curve becomes 'sigmoid' shaped. Middle portion of it is almost a straight line and is suitable for calculations.

Dose response curve is sigmoid shaped.

Figure 1.12 Dose-Response Curve

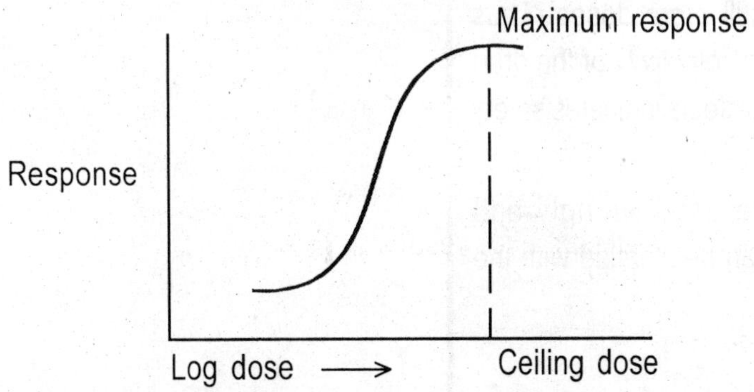

The dose that corresponds to maximum effect is termed as ceiling dose.

The slope of DRC gives an idea about the change in effects when doses are altered. If the slope of DRC is more, a slight change in dose is responsible for large variation in the effect. (Figure1.13 A). If slope of DRC is less, even significant changes in doses may not alter effects significantly. (Figure 1.13 B.).

Steep slope of DRC indicates that small change in a dose alters effects in large proportion.

Figure 1.13 Slope of DRC and effects of drugs

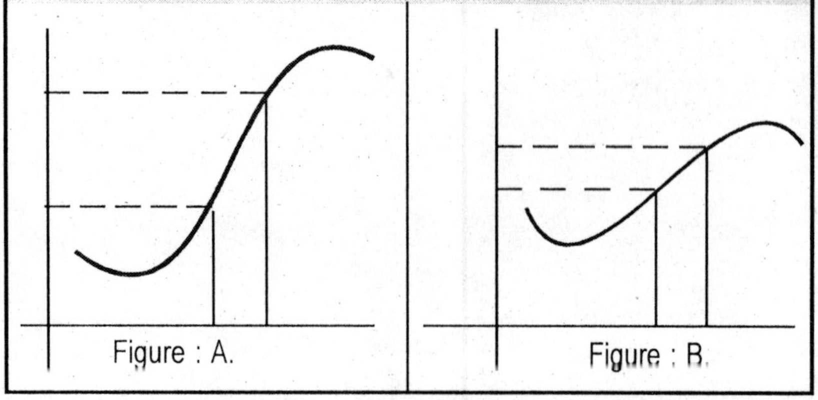

One drug may have different DRCs for different effects and also side effects. If drug A has two effects: one 'increase in heart rate' and second say 'bronchodilatation' and side effect as 'headache'. Then there can be three DRCs.

Figure 1.14 Different DRCs of a same drug

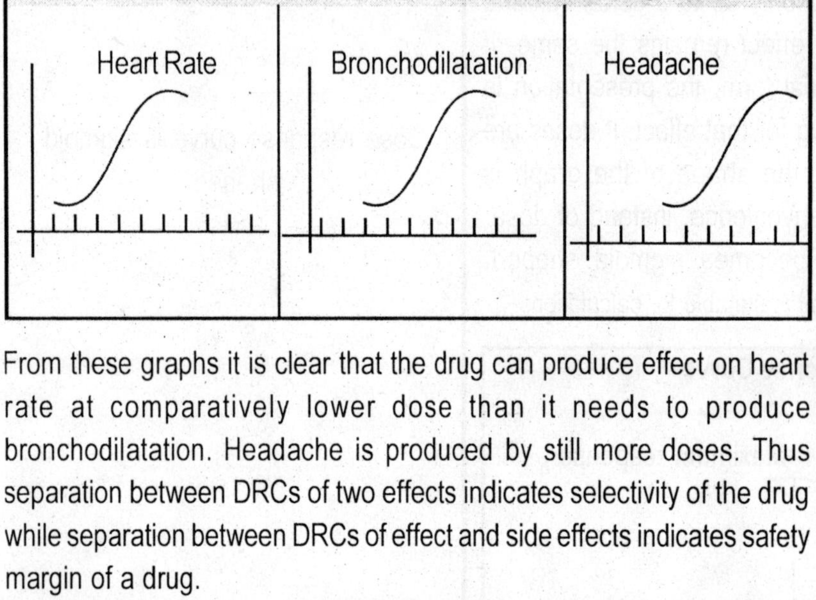

One drug can have different DRCs for different effects and adverse effects.

From these graphs it is clear that the drug can produce effect on heart rate at comparatively lower dose than it needs to produce bronchodilatation. Headache is produced by still more doses. Thus separation between DRCs of two effects indicates selectivity of the drug while separation between DRCs of effect and side effects indicates safety margin of a drug.

Potency and efficacy are two terms that are used wrongly and interchangeably. Difference in these two terms can be clarified with the help of DRC.

Potency

Potency is a weight related term. It is the amount of drug that is required to produce certain effect. It is usually used in comparative sense. Ex. 5 mg of drug A if increases heart rate by 10, and 5 mg of drug B does it by 20, then drug B is more potent than drug A. The potency is reflected by position of DRC along X axis. Shift of DRC along X axis indicates decrease in potency. (Refer Fig. 1.15)

Potency and efficacy are two different terms.

Efficacy or Ceiling Effect

It is the maximum effect that can be produced by a drug. Ex. The same example is continued. The maximum increase in heart rate that can be produced by any dose of drug A is suppose 30, while any dose of drug

B can not increase heart rate by more than 20, then efficacy of drug A is more than B. It is the highest point on the DRC. Thus drug A, compared to drug B is more effective but at the same time less potent. Position of DRC on Y axis reflects efficacy of drug.

In DRC, potency is reflected by displacement on X axis while efficacy on Y axis.

Figure 1.15 Efficacy and potency

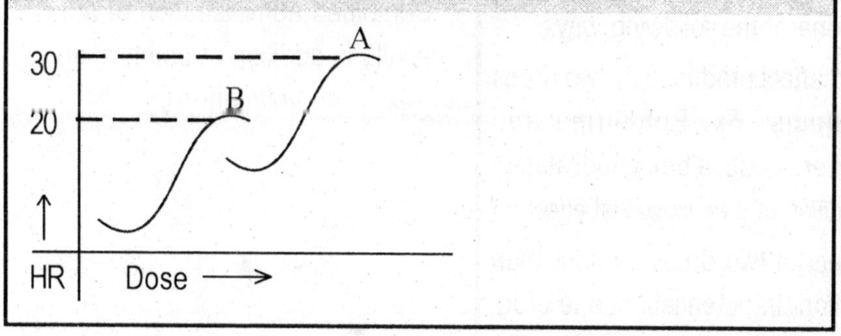

Therapeutic range: It is the range of doses in which a drug can be given safely and effectively. If dose is less than the range, there is no effect and if it is above the range, drug is not that safe.

Therapeutic index: In experimental studies, it is the ratio of: LD 50/ED 50. Where LD 50 is the dose of that drug required to kill 50% of total animals in the study and ED 50 is the dose required to produce desired effect in 50 % of the total animals. In clinical practice therapeutic index is reflected as:

Therapeutic index = Maximum tolerated dose/Minimum effective dose

Or it is the ratio of dose that produces adverse effects in 50% of patients to the dose that produces clinical improvement in 50% of patients. Therapeutic index indicates safety margins. Drugs with high therapeutic index are effective in lower doses and safe in higher doses. It also reflects benefit and risk ratio of drugs. Drugs have multiple effects and side effects. Therefore therapeutic index for each effect and side effect is different. Hence one can't decide one single figure that expresses therapeutic index of drug.

Drugs with high therapeutic index are preferred.

Therapeutic window

In case of some drugs, therapeutic effect of drug is observed within a specific range of doses. Neither doses lesser than that range nor doses more than that can produce effect. The reason for this phenomenon is not clear. This window is observed with drugs like glipizide (antidiabetic) or clonidine (antihypertensive agent). If these agents are not producing clinical effects in patients, either increase in dose or reduction in dose can produce effects.

Combined effects of drugs

Synergism and antagonism

When two or more drugs are administered together, in addition to producing individual effects, they can interfere in each other's action. The net effect is the combined effect of drugs. After co-administration of two drugs there are basically two possibilities.

i) Drugs can work together - (synergism).

ii) Drugs cannot work together - (antagonism).

Synergism

In this type of combined action, two or more drugs when administered together, will have supportive network in one of the following ways -

Combined administration of drugs results in addition or potentiation or antagonism.

1) Addition: In this situation, the combined effect produced by two drugs is equal to addition of individual effects. Ex. Ephedrine and theophylline, when are administered together, produce bronchodilatation by different mechanism and total effect is addition of their individual effects.

2) Potentiation: When the combined effect of two drugs is more than addition of individual effects, it is potentiation. In potentiation, one drug, in addition to producing individual effect, supports action of another. Ex. Sulfamethoxazole and trimethoprim are two bacteriostatic (inhibit multiplication of organisms) antibiotics when given individually but if given together the action is almost bactericidal (kill organisms).

Antagonism: When two drugs are given together and one drug opposes or reduces the effect of another the combined action is termed as antagonism. Depending on the mechanism of opposing the action, antagonism is classified into different types.

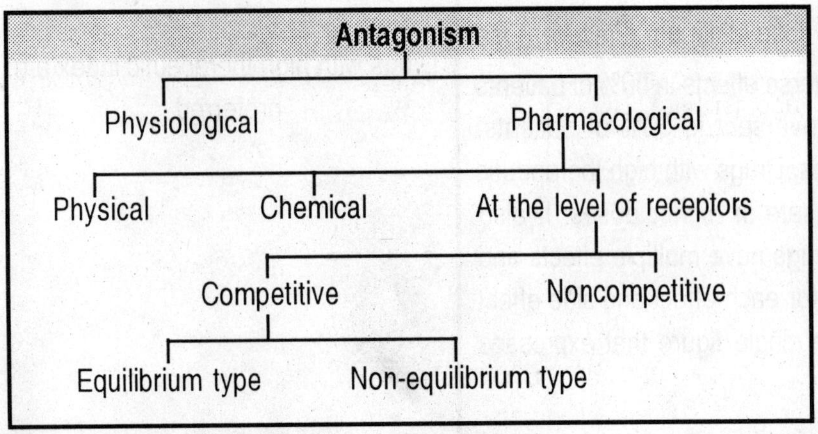

1) In **Physiological antagonism**, two drugs oppose actions of each other by acting at two different locations or by two different mechanisms. EX. In anaphylactic reaction, histamine, through its action on histamine receptors, produces bronchoconstriction and vasodilatation. Adrenaline when is administered as the treatment, acts as physiological antagonist of histamine and through action on adrenergic receptors produces opposite effects i.e. bronchodilatation and vasoconstriction.

Adrenaline and histamine are physiological antagonists

2) In **physical antagonism** action of one drug is reduced by physical interference of another drug. Ex. When any drug is given along with purgatives, increased motility of GI tract (due to purgatives) reduces absorption and then action of the drug.

3) If any chemical reaction is responsible for antagonism, it is **chemical antagonism**. Ex. Chelating agents are the drugs which form chemical complexes with heavy metals and reduce action of heavy metals. (They

are used in metal poisoning)

4) The term **antagonism at receptor level** is used when the site for interference in the action is related to common receptors.

In **competitive antagonism**, both the drugs have affinity for the same receptors and they compete for same receptors. It is of two types.

Competitive-equilibrium type antagonism: Ex. Phenylephrine and prazosin have competitive antagonism of equilibrium type at alpha receptors. Phenylephrine is agonist of α receptor and prazocin is antagonist of α receptor. Both the agents have affinity for alpha receptors. Binding of both of these drugs with receptors is reversible and if concentration of one drug at the receptor site is increased, it displaces the other drug that is bound to receptor.

In competitive antagonism, two or more drugs have affinity for same receptors.

Competitive Non-equilibrium type

Ex. Phenylephrine and phenoxybenzamine have competitive antagonism of Non-equilibrium type. Both the drugs have affinity for alpha receptors; phenylephrine is agonist and phenoxybenzamine is an antagonist of α receptors. The situation is very much similar to prazosin: but here the binding of phenoxybenzamine to alpha receptors is very strong and irreversible. In spite of increasing the concentration of phenylephrine, phenoxybenzamine is not displaced from the receptors.

Noncompetitive: Agonist and antagonist do not have competition for same receptors. Agonist, without competition gets attached to receptors, stimulates receptor but antagonist opposes the action at post receptor level. (not at the site of binding). Ex. Histamine and bicuculine or papaverine.

In noncompetitive antagonism, antagonist acts at post receptor level.

Table 1.7 Competitive and Non competitive antagonism

Competitive (Equilibrium type)	Non competitive
1) Agonist and antagonist are structurally same	No similar structure
2) Both have affinity for the receptor	Only agonist has affinity for the receptor.
3) Competition for binding site	No Competition for binding site
4) If quantity of agonist is increased, it displaces the antagonist and maximum action can be produced but with large dose of agonist	Once antagonist is given; any amount of agonist cannot reverse the action and maximum action is not produced by any dose of agonist.
5. Ex. Phenylephrine and prazosin	Histamine and bicuculine

Figure 1.16 Competitive and non competitive antagonism

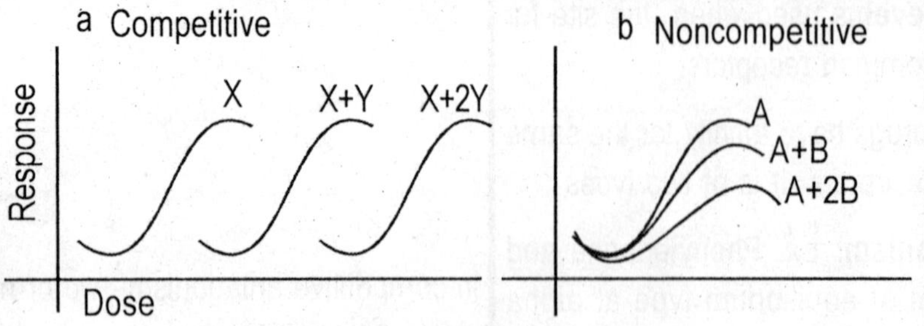

X is agonist, Y is competitive antagonist.
A is agonist, B is noncompetitive antagonist.

In figure 1.16 a, X and Y are competitive antagonists. Graph 1 is DRC of agonist X. Graph 2 is DRC of agonist X after administration of antagonist Y and Graph 3 is DRC of X after administration of high amount of antagonist Y.

In figure 1.16 b, A is an agonist, B is noncompetitive antagonist. Graph 1 is DRC of agonist A. Graph 2 is DRC of agonist A after administration of antagonist B and Graph 3 is DRC of A after administration of high amount of antagonist B.

In equilibrium type when amount of antagonist is increased, more dose of agonist is required to produce maximum response. Hence DRC is shifted to right.

In noncompetitive antagonism, after giving antagonist the maximum action can not be achieved with any amount of agonist and DRC is shifted down. When quantity of antagonist is increased DRC of agonist is still lowered along Y axis.

Competitive (Non-equilibrium type) antagonism behaves partially like competitive equilibrium type antagonism (first 3 point in comparison) and partially like noncompetitive antagonism (fourth point in comparison and alteration in DRC).

DRUG INTERACTIONS

The effects of drugs, when are altered by another drug or food that is co-administered with it, the phenomenon is known as drug-drug or drug-food interaction.

Drug interactions

- Drug-drug interactions
  - Inside body
    - Pharmacokinetic interactions
      - At the levels of
        - Absorption
        - Distribution
        - Metabolism
        - Excretion
    - Pharmacodynamic interactions
  - Outside body
- Drug-food interactions

Drug food interactions

In case of oral administration, if effects of drugs are altered by co-administration of food, the interaction is drug food interaction.

Ex. 1) Milk reduces absorption of tetracycline.

2) Fatty food delays gastric emptying time and alters rate of absorption of any drug that is administered with fatty food.

3) MAO inhibitor drugs, if are administered along with amine containing food, the interaction results in severe hypertension that can result in death.

4) Absorption of many drugs is reduced by food. These drugs are administered on empty stomach.

5) Absorption of some drugs is increased by food.

Some drugs are not taken orally along with food

Drug-drug interaction outside the body

These type of interactions take place when two or more drugs are mixed during intravenous infusion. One drug may get inactivated before it enters into body. Ex. Co-administration of heparin and tetracycline in infusion results in inactivation of tetracycline. Similarly any drug if is administered along with blood or fat solution, it is inactivated.

Drugs can interact outside the body.

Most of the interactions usually take place inside the body. One drug can alter effects of another drug by interfering pharmacokinetics or pharmacodynamics of that drug: (pharmacokinetic interactions and pharmacodynamic interactions).

No drug is mixed in blood during transfusion.

Interaction at the level of absorption

Purgatives increase intestinal motility and do not allow complete absorption. They reduce absorption of many drugs. Antacids reduce absorption of various drugs.

Drugs interact at the levels of absorption, distribution, metabolism, excretion or at the site of action.

Interaction at the level of distribution

Phenylbutazone and tolbutamide share same plasma proteins for protein binding. When these two drugs are administered together, phenylbutazone displaces tolbutamide from protein binding sites. It increases the free tolbutamide available for action. This results in exaggerated actions of tolbutamide (hypoglycemia).

Interaction at the level of metabolism (Refer Page 20).

Phenobarbitone induces the enzymes that are required for metabolism of oral contraceptives. Enhanced metabolism of OC pills results in termination of action and early elimination of drug. Failure of contraception is the result of this interaction.

Interaction at the level of excretion (Refer Page 24).

Probenecid and penicillin are administered together. In kidneys, probenecid is excreted at the place of penicillin and penicillin excretion is reduced. This interaction results in increased duration of action of penicillin.

Pharmacodynamic interactions

In these types of interactions, one drug interferes in the mechanism of action of another drug. Ex. Alcohol alters the effects of antipsychotic drugs or naloxone opposes effects of morphine by blocking opioid receptors (where morphine gets attached). All the examples of pharmacodynamic antagonism come under pharmacodynamic interaction.

Clinical implications of drug interactions

1) Drug interactions are responsible for combined actions like synergism or antagonism. (Refer page 37).

Drug interactions are crucial for drugs having narrow therapeutic range.

2) Two drugs should not be administered together, if one significantly reduces effects of another. Ex. Phenylbutazone is not administered along with OC pills.

3) Sometimes drug interactions are beneficial. Ex. a) Probenecid prolongs the action of penicillin or b) Naloxone can be used in morphine poisoning. c) Adrenaline prolongs the duration of action of local anesthetic agents.

4) Interactions must be carefully watched in case of drugs with narrow therapeutic range. Because slight change in drug concentrations have vast impact on the magnitude of effects and adverse effects. Ex. Digitalis. (Refer page 27).

Some interactions are beneficial and used therapeutically.

5) Sometimes two drugs interact with each other but that interaction clinically is not significant. In these situations co-administration of these agents should not be restricted. Ex. Fluoroquinolones reduce bioavailability of theophylline but the reduction does not have magnitude sufficient for reduction in effects.

Figure 1.17 Interactions at different levels

Steps	Mechanism of interaction
Administration ↓	Inactivation outside body
Absorption ↓	Increased or reduced absorption of drug and food interactions.
Distribution ↓	Displacement from protein binding sites
Action ↓	Antagonism or potentiation
Metabolism ↓	Enzyme induction or inhibition
Elimination	Increase or decrease in elimination of drugs

Fixed dose combinations (FDCs)

Various clinical situations demand administration of more than one drugs. In that case, drugs can be administered together either in two different formulation (co-administration) or in one single formulation. Fixed dose combination contains at least two drugs in single formulation.

Fixed dose combination contains two or more drugs in one formulation.

Advantages

i) Improved compliance: FDCs reduce the number of administrations and improve compliance; e.g. In common cold, rather than taking 9 tablets/day (3/day of antipyretic, 3/day of decongestant and 3/day of antihistaminic), FDC of analgesic + antihistaminic + antipyretic allows only 3 administrations.

Major advantage of FDC is improved compliance; but FDCs have many disadvantages also.

ii) Additional effects: FDCs of estrogen and progesterone in oral contraceptives have synergistic action.

iv) Reduction in adverse effects: FDC of L-Dopa and carbidopa allows administration of less amount of L-Dopa and side effects are reduced. (Refer page 18).

v) Cost of treatment is reduced by FDCs.

Limitations

i) Drugs with different frequencies of administration or different durations of treatment can not be combined in FDC.

ii) Drugs that have negative interaction with each other can't be combined.

iii) If one of the drugs in FDCs demands dose adjustment or early termination, it is not possible with FDC.

iv) If any ingredient in FDC has food interaction or if it is contraindicated in some situation; the whole FDC is contraindicated.

v) In case of improvement in disease, the agent in FDC that has provided the effects is not known.

Compliance

A drug is not effective if it is not taken

A drug is not effective if it is not taken. Compliance is the patient's adherence to the treatment schedule. This is a comparatively neglected issue in clinical practice but is very crucial.

Following factors reduce compliance -

i) Multi-prescription: Prescription of too many drugs.

ii) Increased frequency of administration (like qid or more)

iii) Prolonged duration of treatment

iv) Complicated instruction: Ex. Drugs should not be taken along with the food. Such instructions reduce freedom of administration and reduce compliance.

Complicated schedules and instructions reduce compliance.

v) Adverse effects of drugs, if are severe or more, patients avoid taking drugs.

vi) Nature of the disease: If administration of drug does not provide immediate relief, patients postpone or forget to take the drug. Ex. Compliance for pain killer in acute pain will always be more than that for vitamin capsules.

vii) Personality of patient: Non cooperative patients, having no belief in doctor or medication or patients with impaired memory are prone for noncompliance.

Compliance is measured primarily by proper history taking, checking containers or empty foils. Recently some electronic devices are used in developed countries.

Consequences of noncompliance are hardly benign. They include:

i) Increased morbidity and mortality

ii) Increased cost : of another drug course and doctor fees

iii) Incomplete antibacterial treatment results in development of resistance for that antibacterial agent.

Noncompliance for antibiotics produces resistant organisms.

Placebo

Actual meaning of word placebo is 'shall I please'. It is the drug that is given to please the patient. Placebo is a pharmacologically inert substance as far as that disease is concerned. It has no effect on the natural course of disease but it provides only psychological relief to the patient. The effect of placebo depends on following factors:

1) Personality of patient: Different personalities show different reactions to placebos.

i) Placebo reactors (usually extrovert individuals) show good response to placebo medication.

ii) Placebo nonreactors (usually introvert individuals) do not respond to placebo medication.

iii) Negative reactors: Placebo doesn't produce desired effects but only adverse effects in these patients.

2) Type of disease: Psychiatric disorders or chronic disorders respond well to placebos.

3) Route and appearance of placebo: Colorful tablets or injectables have more placebo effect.

Indications: Placebo is used when:

i) Doctor is not sure about diagnosis,

ii) Alternative treatment is not available,

iii) Patient and disease demand some treatment,

iv) Placebos are used in clinical trials as dummy medications to compare results of active drugs.

TOXICOLOGY

It is the branch of pharmacology that deals with undesired harmful effects of drugs. Almost every drug administration is associated with some undesired effects. The Benefit and Risk ratio of drug decides the acceptability of a drug. Ex. Severe harmful effects of anticancer drugs are acceptable because the benefit is almost life. Nobody will accept similar type of undesired effects for a drug which is useful in common cold. Some of the undesired effects can be explained on the basis of pharmacological actions while some are not. Therefore, absence of pharmacological reasoning does not rule out the causativity. It is the

Severe adverse effects are acceptable; if benefits are significant.

confirmation of certainty that decides the relation between drug and undesired effects. When this relation is established, there are following possibilities.

i) Accept the risk and use the drug.
ii) Restricted use of drug
iii) Searching for new derivatives with same effects and less side effects
iv) Withdrawn from the market

Side effects: These are minor and predictable undesired harmful effects. They are explainable on the basis of pharmacology. Ex. Pharmacological effect of insulin is reduction in blood sugar levels. Insulin can cause side effect hypoglycemia as the extension of its pharmacological action.

Adverse effects: These are undesired harmful effects that are more serious (compared to side effects) and may or may not have explainable pharmacological basis. Adverse effects are produced by therapeutic dose range and usually demand withdrawal of the drug or reduction in its dose. Ex. Severe constipation caused by codeine is an adverse effect that demands change of drug or reduction in dose.

Adverse effects are produced with therapeutic doses while toxic effects with excess doses.

Toxicity: Toxicity refers to undesired harmful effects due to excess dose i.e. more than therapeutic dose. Ex. Overdose of paracetamol causes hepatotoxicity. If metabolizing capacity of body is impaired, drug that is administered in therapeutic doses is not sufficiently metabolised. This accumulation results in toxicity with therapeutic dose.

Secondary adverse effects: These adverse effects are produced as the indirect consequences of drugs. Ex. If antibiotics are taken for a long time gastrointestinal flora is altered and there are chances of superinfections.

Iatrogenic disorders: 'Iatros' means a physician. Iatrogenic disorders are the diseases that are caused by drugs or doctors. Some side effects are expected of all drugs. Whether they are acceptable or not depends on individual judgement and scientific back up. The issue is little subjective and controversial. But in most of the situations it is lack of knowledge or negligence that is responsible for these Iatrogenic disorders. Before calling a certain disorder as 'Iatrogenic', definite correlation between drug and the disorder must be established. These disorders have medicolegal importance. Ex. Antipsychotics can cause retinopathy. Non steroidal antiinflammatory drugs like aspirin, ibuprofen, after long-term use, produce peptic ulcers. Amikacin develops deafness and long term steroid therapy results in osteoporosis.

Drugs or doctors produce iatrogenic disorders.

Intolerance: There are lot of controversies in defining the term intolerance: The simplest interpretation of the term intolerance suggests reduced capacity of a body to tolerate a drug. Body may not tolerate specific quantity (quantitative intolerance) or may not tolerate any quantity (qualitative intolerance: idiosyncracy and hypersensitivity).

Quantitative intolerance: It is exaggerated quantitative response to therapeutic dose of a drug by an individual. Ex. Drug in a dose of 5 mg normally increases heart rate by 10. In an individual who has intolerance, the same dose will increase heart rate by 40.

Drug intolerance can be quantitative (conventional intolerance) or qualitative (idiosyncrasy and hypersensitivity)

Idiosyncracy: The word 'Idiosyncracy' is coined from three words, viz, idios (self), syn (with) and krasis (to mingle). Idiosyncracy is occurrence of qualitative abnormal effects of drug in an individual. It is not the exaggeration of the normal pharmacological effects. The reason usually is genetic, but sometimes no genetic or pharmacological basis can explain the idiosyncratic reaction.

Pharmacogenetics

Pharmacogenetics is a science that deals with effects of drugs, which are altered by genetic structure of an individual. A variety of genetic alterations are proved to have effects on the actions of drugs.

1) Genetic deficiency of G6PD (Glucose 6 Phosphate Dehydrogenase): G6PD is a substance in the body, which is a source of NADPH. NADPH maintains glutathione in erythrocytes in reduced form which further maintains hemoglobin in reduced form. This is essential for intact cell membranes of erythrocytes. In an individual who has genetic deficiency of G6PD, if erythrocytes are exposed to oxidant drugs like dapsone, primaquine or quinolones, there is oxidative destruction of RBCs that leads to hemolysis. In normal individual these drugs never produce this effect.

2) Acetylation status: Acetylation is one of the reactions involved in metabolism of some drugs. Rate of acetylation is governed genetically. Depending on this rate individuals are classified into slow acetylators and fast acetylators. Some drug can produce different effects in these two classes of individuals. Ex. INH, after acetylation, is converted into a metabolite acetylhydrazine. In fast acetylators the metabolism is faster and there is collection of acetylhydrazine which has hepatotoxicity. In slow acetylators, the metabolite is slowly formed ; but there is accumulation of unmetabolized INH. INH interferes in pyridoxin functions and results in peripheral neuropathy. Thus two genetically different classes produce different side effects for the same drug: fast acetylators experience hepatotoxicity and slow acetylators show neuropathies.

Genetic structure of an individual can alter effects of drugs

3) Psuedocholinesterase deficiency: Succinylcholine is a drug used in surgeries as a skeletal muscle relaxant. Enzyme pseudocholinesterase is required for termination of action of succinylcholine. Genetic deficiency of this enzyme prolongs the action of succinylcholine. Prolonged relaxation of respiratory muscles produces breathlessness for a long time. This genetic abnormality is termed as *scoline apnea.*

5) Resistance to some antibiotics or tolerance to some anticoagulants is also genetically governed.

Some idiosyncratic reactions do not have genetic basis. Ex. Vascular collapse after quinidine has neither genetic nor pharmacological basis.

Hypersensitivity

It is not the exaggerated sensitivity to a drug; as the word suggests. Hypersensitivity is an exaggerated immunological response to drug or excipients. This is a qualitative response and not related to amount of drug. Many times body reacts immunologically for a variety of drugs; but hypersensitivity refers only to the reaction which is undesired and harmful.

Hypersensitivity has got nothing to do with the quantity of drug.

Basis for hypersensitivity

First exposure to the drug. (drug acts as antigen or foreign body)

↓

Sensitization of body. (Antibodies are produced against drug or T lymphocytes are synthesized against that drug).

↓

Second exposure to the same drug.

↓

Immunological reaction. (between drug and antibody or drug and T lymphocytes).

↓

Harmful effects.

These are immunological reactions and are observed after second exposure to the drug.

Hypersensitivity reactions are classified on the basis of immunological reactions: Type I, II, III and IV. Details of the mechanisms of these types of hypersensitivity reactions are discussed on page 48 and 49.

Clinical implications

1) Before prescribing any drug, the doctor must get the history of hypersensitivity for the drugs that are to be prescribed. Known hypersensitivity is contraindication for all drugs.

2) If hypersensitivity is present without the history of prior administration of drug, it does not rule out the diagnosis of hypersensitivity. Patient may get sensitized through drug in breast milk or dairy products (If the drug is administered to animals).

3) Sensitization tests can be conducted in case of drugs that have high incidence of allergic reactions Ex. Penicillins.

4) Treatment of hypersensitivity reactions is crucial and it largely depends on the type and gravity of the reaction. The drug is immediately discontinued. Depending on the type of reactions, antihistamines, adrenaline, aminophylline or steroids are used in allergic reactions.

Type I. Anaphylaxis or Immediate hypersensitivity reactions	Type II. Cytolytic hypersensitivity or cytotoxic reactions
First exposure to a drug ↓ Sensitisation ↓ Generation of IgE antibodies ↓ Antibodies get fixed to mast cells ↓ Second exposure to drug ↓ Antigen (Drug) Antibody reaction ↓ Release of histamine, PAF, PGs leukotrienes from mast cells ↓ Vasodilatation Bronchoconstriction Itching Edema Ex. Allergy to penicillin (PAF: Platelet Activating Factor) PGs: Prostaglandins	First exposure to drug ↓ Drug gets combined with some cell components (proteins) and the complex acts as an antigen ↓ Sensitisation ↓ Generation of IgG and IgM antibodies ↓ Antibodies are attached to different cells ↓ Second exposure to drug ↓ Antigen (drug + cell component) Antibody reaction ↓ Destruction of cells to which antibodies are attached ↓ Hemolysis Agranulocytosis Thrombocytopenia Aplastic anemia Ex. Penicillin induced anemia.

Hypersensitivity Type I / II / III reactions are antibody mediated while type IV is cells mediated.

Type III Hypersensitivity or Arthus reaction	Type IV or delayed hypersensitivity reactions.
First exposure to drug ↓ Sensitisation ↓ Generation of IgG antibodies ↓ Antibodies float freely in the blood ↓ Second exposure to the drug ↓ Antigen (Drug) Antibody reaction ↓ Formation of complex of antigen and antibody ↓ Complexes get attached to capillaries and produce endothelial damage ↓ Release of lysosomes ↓ Vascular inflammatory response, rash, serum sickness, fever, arthralgia, lymphadenopathy Ex. Phenylbutazone, sulfonamides	First exposure to a drug ↓ Sensitisation ↓ Generation of new T lymphocytes with receptor for that drug ↓ Second exposure to the drug ↓ Antigen (Drug) gets attached to sensitised T lymphocytes ↓ Release of lymphokines ↓ Granulocytes are attracted ↓ Contact dermatitis or granuloma formation Ex. Topical antibiotics, local anesthetic agents.

Penicillins, sulfonamides, tetracyclines, local anesthetics etc. are some of the common drugs that can produce various hypersensitivity reactions.

Anaphylaxis is characterized by bronchoconstriction and shock. Management of anaphylactic reaction is crucial and is life saving. It involves following steps;

i) Keeping airway patent

ii) Adrenaline 0.5 ml of 1:1000 IM or 3-5 ml of 1:10,000 IV (It reverses hypotension and bronchoconstriction) It is a drug of choice

iii) Fluid level correction.

iv) Sympathomimetic agents like noradrenaline or dopamine

v) 100 mg IV hydrocortisone

vi) Antihistaminics, bronchodilators as per requirement.

· 'Hypersensitivity for a drug' is an absolute contraindication for that drug.

Pseudoallergic reactions

Symptoms and overall appearance of clinical picture in these reactions are very much similar to allergic reactions. But immunological reaction is not there. These are nonimmunologic reactions. The reasons may be genetic. Ex. Reactions to thiopentone, morphine or bronchial asthma induced by aspirin.

Pseudoallergic reactions have no immunological basis.

Teratogenicity

Terratos is a monster. Administration of a few drugs during pregnancy results in birth of monster like baby. Teratogenicity term refers to undesired harmful effects of a drug on the fetus when the drug is administered to mother during pregnancy. Such drug may not have similar type of adverse effects on the body of mother. The reasons for teratogenicity are attributed to chemical nature of the drug and to the placental barrier which exposes fetus to almost all drugs that are administered to mother. They can have direct effect on the fetal cells or can alter vascular supply of the fetus and produce harmful effects.

Teratogenic drugs may not be harmful for mothers.

Pregnancy is detected only one month after the conception and no drug restriction is possible before that. After that, up to 2 months is the period of organogenesis and from 2-9 months there is the period of growth and development. Administration of teratogenic drug in first two months usually develops structural abnormalities while administration of such drugs afterwards results in developmental abnormalities Ex. Thalidomide crisis had a lot of contribution in development of norms related to use of drugs in pregnancy. Administration of thalidomide in pregnancies resulted in phocomelia (sealed limbs) in neonates. The drug was banned after that episode.

Table 1.8 Teratogenic effects of drugs

Drugs used in pregnancy	Abnormalities in fetus
1) Phenytoin	Fetal hydantoin syndrome: microcephaly, cleft palate, hypoplastic nails etc.
2) Alcohol in first trimester	Retardation of mental and physical growth
3) Tetracycline	Abnormal teeth and decreased growth of bones
4) Testosterone	Masculinization of fetus.

Clinical applications

1) Known teratogenic drugs are contraindicated in pregnancy.

2) Finding safety of drugs in pregnancy is not an easy job. In clinical trials pregnant females are usually excluded. So data regarding safe use of a drug in pregnancy is difficult to get. It needs a long period before data gets collected. The drug is used only when the risk of using drug in pregnancy is much less as compared to probable benefits. Depending on this data and animal studies drugs are classified into various categories. These categories are used as guidelines for

administration of drug in pregnancy.

3) Some drugs are not contraindicated in pregnancies but are not proved as safe; Use of such drugs in pregnant females depends on subjective judgement of benefit and risk ratio.

Tolerance

Tolerance is requirement of more amount to produce certain effect.

Concept of tolerance can be explained in easiest possible way with the example of effect of alcohol. Specific quantity of alcohol produces a certain effect in Central Nervous System. After periodic consumption of alcohol the same quantity of alcohol can not produce the same effect. The effect is reduced. To get the same effect, one has to consume more amount of alcohol. This is development of tolerance for alcohol. Drugs also follow similar rules. Sometimes tolerance is observed even when drug is administered for the first time.

By definition tolerance is the requirement of more amount of drug to produce specific response. Tolerance can be natural or acquired.

Natural tolerance has genetic basis while acquired tolerance is due to exposure.

i) Natural tolerance: It is the presence of tolerance without prior exposure to the drug. Effects of drugs in a few individuals or few species are less in magnitude from the very first exposure to drug. Ex. Some individuals require more amount of anticoagulants as compared to normal therapeutic doses. The reasons are usually genetic.

ii) Acquired tolerance: It is the development of tolerance after a prolonged or rapid or excessive use of drugs.

Mechanisms for development of acquired tolerance

a) Down-regulation of receptors: It is the decrease in number and sensitivity of receptors for an agonist after prolonged exposure to it. (Refer page 33).

b) Internalization of receptor: After prolonged exposure to agonists some receptors are taken inside the cell and they remain unavailable for action.

c) Enzyme induction: Alcohol induces hepatic microsomal enzymes that are required for its own metabolism. So long term use of alcohol results in faster metabolism and elimination and reduced action of alcohol. (Refer Page 20).

d) Tachyphylaxis: It is the development of tolerance after repeated administrations of a drug. Ex. Ephedrine stimulates release of stored noradrenaline from the nerve endings. After repeated administrations of ephedrine, the store of noradrenaline is exhausted and effect of ephedrine is reduced.

Tachyphylaxis: Rapid development of tolerance.

Clinical implications of tolerance:

Tolerance for effects may not be associated with that for adverse effects.

i) Previous prolonged exposure to drug can produce clinical effects that are less than what are expected

ii) Development of tolerance when demands increase in doses, decision is not very easy. Because tolerance for effect may not be associated with tolerance for side effects.

iii) Cross tolerance: If prolonged use of one drug results in development of tolerance for another drug, it is cross tolerance for another drug. Such two drugs are usually similar in either structure or in function. Ex. Prolonged exposure to barbiturates results in development of tolerance for hypnotic agents.

Cross tolerance: exposure to one drug: tolerance for another.

Pseudo tolerance: From the prehistoric period, poisons are consumed regularly and in small quantities to develop tolerance against them. This type of logic is not scientifically proved.

Dependence

Some drugs are consumed just to get pleasure. There is no clinical indication for these drugs. This nonmedical, unindicated self administration of drugs is called as '*drug abuse*'. Abuse can result in dependence for that drug. Prolonged medical use of drugs also can result in dependence. Dependence is a state which arises due to repeated, periodic or continuous administration of a drug. It is initially characterized by a desire for the drug, then need and then compulsion to take that drug. Dependence is associated with withdrawal reactions. Withdrawal reactions are the undesired effects that are observed if the drug is not administered.

Dependence can be physical or psychological.

Dependence can be psychological or physical.

Psychological dependence: This dependence has following criteria:
i) Patient thinks that the drug is required for psychological well being,
ii) Withdrawal effects are mainly associated with emotional problems. Ex. Tobacco withdrawal in tobacco dependence is associated with mood disturbances. Laxative dependence also has a major psychological component.

Physical dependence: Criteria for physical dependence are:
i) Neuroadaptational changes take place in the body due to prolonged administration of the drug. Neuroadaptational change: Ex. Prolonged external administration of morphine results in reduced secretion of morphine like substances (opioids) in the body. Sudden withdrawal of external morphine exposes the body to sudden lack of these opioids. Ex. Morphine withdrawal is associated with irritability, insomnia, muscle spasms. Psychological component can not be separated in physical dependence.

Neuroadaptational changes are responsible for withdrawal reactions.

ii) Drug administration is required for physical activities.
iii) Withdrawal of drug results in physical problems.

Predisposing factors for dependence

1) Dependence potential of drugs: Opioids, amphetamines, alcohol, barbiturates, nicotine, caffeine are some drugs that have dependence potential. Mood modifying actions of drugs contribute largely in

development of dependence.

2) Easy access to drugs: especially in health workers.

3) Unstable life style, stress, family tensions make one vulnerable for abuse and dependence

4) Influence of social circle.

Clinical implications of dependence

i) Dependence, on drugs leads to tolerance for the drugs and reduced effects of drugs.

ii) Dependence after a certain limit, interferes substantially in personal, social and legal life and is termed as addiction. Drug addiction leads to various physical and psychological disorders. It is one of the reasons of suicides.

Treatment of drug dependence : Drug dependence should be carefully treated with two basic objectives. One is to prevent unindicated consumption and second to prevent or treat withdrawal reactions. Steps in the treatment of dependence are as follows. -

i) Gradual withdrawal of the drug,

ii) Replacement therapy: A drug with parallel and controlled effects can be used as replacement. Ex. benzodiazepines are used in alcohol dependence when alcohol is gradually withdrawn.

iii) Symptomatic treatment of pain, cramps etc.

iv) Psychotherapy,

v) If drug dependence does not affect social life significantly and withdrawal effects are serious enough, restricted amount of drug (on which patient is dependent) is administered as a therapy.

Treatment of dependence:
Prevent consumption
Treat withdrawal reactions

Carcinogenicity

It is the capacity of a drug to produce cancers in human body. Usually long term treatment results in carcinogenicity but nitrosamines are known to be carcinogenic in single dose.

Various mechanisms are responsible for carcinogenicity of drugs.

i) Some drugs cause mutations and activate oncogens.

ii) Some drugs suppress immunity and produce cancers.

iv) Hormonal imbalance caused by some drugs results in development of cancers.

Carcinogenic drugs include griseofulvin, estrogens, omeprazole and above all some anticancer drugs are carcinogenic.

FACTORS AFFECTING ACTIONS OF DRUGS

Suppose 5 mg tablet of drug A increases heart rate by 10 in one person. Same tablet if is given to another person, heart rate may increase by 15. Same tablet if is administered by sublingual route, heart rate may increase by 25. The same amount of drug if is given by intramuscular route, heart rate may not increase but altogether different action can be produced. In brief pharmacology is not mathematics. There are lot of variables. Human body is not a machine and there are various factors that can modify the actions of drugs. Before prescribing any drug, these factors must be considered. Knowledge, judgement and experience in the medicinal field give insight into these factors. It is due to these factors, prescriptions of all doctors for the same disorders are not the same and it is due to these factors, computers cannot replace doctors.

Pharmacology is not mathematics; effects of drugs are not like simple calculations.

For sake of convenience, these factors are classified into two types: Factors related to patient or host and factors related to administration.

Table 1.9 Factors affecting actions of drugs

Factors related to Host	Factors related to administration
1)Race	1) Route of administration
2) Genetic factors	2) Place and time of administration
3) Body size and weight.	3) Co-administration with another drug
4) Age	4) Co-administration with food
5) Sex	5) Previous exposure to drug: tolerance or cumulative effects.
6) Psychological status	
7) Disease status	

Race: Some races react differently to some drugs. Ex. Indian population is resistant to thiacetazone, an antitubercular drug. The black hypertensive population has low plasma renin activity and higher plasma volume as compared to the white and they respond better to diuretics.

Genetic factors: Genetic variation in individual person sometimes is responsible for alteration in the effects of a drug. The issue has already been discussed in details (Refer Page 46). Ex. Metabolizing capacity of INH is governed genetically. Slow acetylators will have peripheral neuropathy as the side effect of INH (due to accumulation of free INH) and fast acetylators will have hepatotoxicity as the side effect (due to accumulation of hepatotoxic metabolite).

Body size and weight: Variations in weight and body surface area alter distribution and hence the actions of drugs. Individuals with more body size or weight obviously demand more drug to produce certain effects. Ideally all doses of drugs should be described on the basis of mg/kg base but this is not practicable. Each individual will require different dose. Then formulation of drugs in specific strengths will be impossible. To avoid this inconvenience standard doses that are generally suitable are used clinically. Guidelines for individual doses according to weight or surface are roughly defined as:

$$\text{Individual dose} = \frac{\text{Body wt (kg)}}{70} \times \text{Average adult dose}$$

$$\text{Individual dose} = \frac{\text{Body surface area (m}^2\text{)}}{1.7} \times \text{Average adult dose}$$

Age: Two extremities, children and aged, react differently to drugs. Children should not be treated as compressed adults. Body size and body weight are not the only factors that differentiate children from adults. Compared to adults, a child reacts differently to drugs at various levels. Table 1.10 explains why children need special concern in pharmacology.

Children are not compressed adults.

Table 1.10 Children and effects of drugs

Level	Variation in children: (compared to adults)
Formulation	Solid forms are not easily acceptable
Absorption	Skin is thinner so more cutaneous absorption. Rectal absorption is faster. Suppositories are preferred. Muscle mass less, slow intramuscular absorption. Low gastric acidity: altered absorption
Distribution	Less body weight and body surface area: less volume for distribution. Percentage of water content is more, which affects distribution. Children require more quantity of theophylline (wt/wt.) compared to adults.
Metabolism	Underdeveloped enzymatic systems reduce metabolism drugs and increase accumulation and toxicity.
Excretion	Slow elimination
Alteration in dose	$\frac{\text{Age}}{\text{Age} + 12}$ x adult dose or on the basis of mg/kg.
Adverse effects	Drugs like quinolones or tetracycline may interfere in development of bones or joints only in children.

Geriatric population also has different variations that are responsible for altered actions.

1) Reduced lean body mass: Less drug distribution
2) Decreased water content in the body: Altered distribution
3) Decreased metabolizing capacity: Accumulation and toxicity
4) Reduced capacity of nephrons: Accumulation and toxicity
5) Down-regulation of receptors: Reduced effects of drugs
6) Multiple prescriptions in elderly population lead to drug interactions.
7) Elderly population has intolerance for drugs like diuretics.

All these variations affect effects and adverse effects of drugs in geriatric population and proper precautions must be taken.

Sex: Males and females react differently to some drugs. Following are the situations where sex interferes in pharmacology.

Table 1.11 Sex and effects of drugs

Hormonal status	Administration of male sex hormones can improve impotence in males but produces virilism (hair growth) in females. Oral contraceptives are only administered in females.
Adverse effects	Gynecomastia is an adverse effect of cimetidine that is present only in males.
Pregnancy	In pregnancy, drugs may react differently due to altered (i) GI motility, (ii) water fat proportion, and (iii) renal blood flow. Additionally teratogenicity restricts use of some drugs in females. Ex. Tetracyclines.
Breast feeding	Excretion of some drugs in breast milk restricts their use in lactating mothers.

Psychological status

Actions of drugs are affected by two psychological factors.

i) Personality: Different personalities may react differently to different antipsychotic drugs, or extrovert individuals react better to placebo.

ii) Emotional status at the time of administration; In highly elated state of mind hypnotic drugs like diazepam will act differently as compared to depressed state.

Sometimes, emotional status at the time of administration alters effects of drugs.

Disease status: Two types of diseases can alter effects of drugs.

i) Diseases for which the drug is administrated, and

ii) Associated diseases. The way different diseases can affect actions of drugs are explained below.

Hepatic and renal disorders demand alterations is dosages

Table 1.12 Diseases and effects of drugs

Diseases	Effects on the drugs
Diarrhoea or increased GI motility	Reduced absorption time and effect
Muscular atrophy	Decreased circulation in muscles and reduced absorption of drug after IM injection
Surgical resection of intestines	Reduced area available for absorption.
Liver disorders	Effects are different due to i) Altered metabolism of drugs. ii) Absence of first pass effect. iii) Prodrug may not get converted into active form
Renal disorders	Reduced clearances: accumulation of drugs. Proper dose adjustment for drugs like cephalexin or ciprofloxacin is required in renal disorders.
Inflammed meninges	Improved absorption of drugs through blood brain barrier.

Factors associated with administration

Route: Some drugs, when are administered by different routes produce different actions; qualitatively and quantitatively.

Quantitative difference: Subcutaneous administration of insulin reduces blood sugar levels within physiological limits. The same amount given intravenously may cause death due to convulsions.

Qualitative difference: Magnesium sulfate, if given orally, acts as purgative and if applied topically reduces swelling. If it is administered injectably it reduces blood pressure.

Place and time of administration: Circadian rhythm interferes with the action of drug. Ex. Hypnotics will act better if they are administered just before regular sleeping time. Not only the time but the place of drug administration also matters, though very rarely. At high altitudes, reduced atmospheric oxygen may retard metabolism of some drugs.

Concurrent administration of another drug

(Refer page 40: Drug-drug interactions)

Concurrent administration of food

(Refer page 41: Drug-food interactions)

Previous exposure to a drug

Prolonged previous exposure to a drug results in tolerance which is responsible for unexpected reduction in the action of a drug. (Refer page 51). Previous exposure to drug may result in accumulation of drug in the body. Administration of subsequent normal dose produces toxicity in these situations. Drugs like lead or digitalis are commonly accumulated in the body.

Routes of administration

Drugs are administered by different routes. Change in route of administration of drug not only alters the magnitude of effect of the drug but also the action itself. Ex. Magnesium sulfate, if given by oral route acts as purgative while applied topically reduces swelling and administered injectably reduces blood pressure. Therefore selection of route is not as simple as one thinks.

Sometimes drug produces altogether different effects by different routes.

Routes of administration of drugs basically are classified as

i) Local route: Drug administered by this route is not absorbed or minimally absorbed in the circulation and acts at the site of administration:

ii) Systemic route: When drug is administered by systemic route, it is absorbed in systemic circulation and the drug acts all over the body. Administration through same routes, sometimes has local effects, while sometimes systemic effects.

Local route: drug acts at the site of administration.

Systemic route: drug acts all over body.

Table 1.13 Local routes of administration

Local routes
1) Skin: cream, lotions etc. In skin infections or eczema
2) Mucus membranes: mouth gel (oral sores), eye drops (infections), urethra (urethritis).
3) Rectal steroids in ulcerative colitis
4) Pulmonary: terbutaline inhalation
5) Intracardiac: adrenaline in cardiac arrest
6) Intraarticular: steroids in joints
7) Intraarterial: anticancer drugs in arteries supplying tumor

Table 1.14 Systemic routes of administration

Systemic routes
1) Oral: tablets, capsules, liquids
2) Rectal: antibiotic suppositories
3) Pulmonary: inhalational anesthetic agents.
4) Sublingual: keeping tablet under tongue: nitroglycerine
5) Cutaneous: promoting absorption through skin
6) Nasal: (not pulmonary): insulin is absorbed through nasal mucosa.
Injections
7) Intradermal - in the skin.
8) Subcutaneous - below skin.
9) Intramuscular - in muscle.
10) Intravenous - in vein.
11) Intraperitoneal - in peritoneal cavity.

Same route can be used for local or systemic effects.

Sometimes same route can be utilized for local application or systemic administration. Various factors are crucial in deciding proper route for administration of drugs. Following are some factors that must be considered before deciding the route of administration. Advantages and limitations of various routes can be predicted by applying these factors to different routes.

Table 1.15 Factors affecting routes of administration	
I Factors related to drugs	
Chemical nature Alteration in bioavailability Therapeutic range Drug interactions Adverse effects	
II Factors related to administration	**III Factors related to patient**
Rapidity of action Reversibility Technical expertise Acceptability	Age Consciousness Disease status Compliance Cost

Factors related to drugs

1) Chemical nature: Some drugs can't be administered by some routes. Ex. Insulin, if given orally, is destroyed in gastrointestinal tract. Hence it is given by subcutaneous route.

2) Alteration in bioavailability: If a drug undergoes first pass effect then its bioavailability is reduced if given orally. (Refer Page 21). Hence it is administered by different routes. Ex. Nitroglycerine by sublingual route.

3) Drugs with narrow therapeutic range: Slight reduction in concentration of these agents leads to loss of effects and slight increase in concentration produces severe adverse effects. In such situations route that offers accuracy is preferred.

4) Drug interactions: If a drug has significant interaction with food or other drugs taken orally, any other route (except oral) is preferred.

5) Adverse effects: If a drug is capable of producing side effects at the site of administration, alternative route must be preferred. Ex. If oral iron produces severe GI intolerance, iron is administered by IM route. Some drugs produce pain and necrosis at the site of injection.

Some adverse effects are associated with specific routes

Factors related to administration

1) Rapidity of action: In emergency situation rapid initiation of action is crucial. IV route is preferred in these conditions. EX. IV streptokinase in myocardial infarction.

2) Reversibility: Accidental administration of excess quantity, sometimes, demands withdrawal of a drug. Ex. After sublingual administration of nitroglycerine, if there are signs of overdose, the tablet kept under the tongue is thrown out.

3) Supervision and technical expertise : Routes like intravenous route require technical skills while oral drugs are self administered.

4) Accuracy : For drugs with narrow therapeutic range, precise amount should be administered. The exact amount may not be achieved by oral route. So injectable routes are preferred.

5) Acceptability for administration : Bitter test after oral administration or pain after IM injection may demand change in the route of administration to improve compliance.

Factors related to patients

1) Age: Oral administration of tablets is not suitable for neonates. Injectable or rectal routes are preferred.

2) Consciousness: Routes that require voluntary participation of patients can't be used in unconscious patients. Ex. Oral route.

Oral administration is not possible in unconscious patients.

3) Disease status: Muscular dystrophy may limit IM use of drugs or vomiting may limit oral administration.

4) Compliance: In case of noncooperative patients oral route is not dependable and supervised therapy is essential.

5) Cost: The same amount of same drug by different routes needs different costs. It includes cost of formulation, accessories (syringes- etc.) and charges of administration (in case of injectable routes).

Each route of administration, when is correlated with these factors, gives idea about the advantages or limitations of that route. Oral and IV routes are discussed in details.

Different local routes of administrations are already discussed in table 1.13. The major advantage with local administration is availability of drug precisely at the site of actions. Additional advantage is absence of absorption (or minimal absorption) in systemic circulation, which reduces undesired effects of drugs. In case of topical route the advantage of easy application is compensated by a disadvantage; lack of accuracy. Exact quantity of topically applied drug is difficult to measure.

Oral route of administration

It is the most commonly used route of administration and various formulations like tablets, capsules, syrups, etc. are administered by this route. Orally administered drugs are absorbed into circulation through blood vessels of GI tract.

Advantages of oral route

Easy administration

No supervision or expertise is required

Cost: Oral formulations are comparatively cheap

Reversibility : In case of oral overdose vomiting can be induced or gastric lavage is possible.

Limitations of oral route

Consciousness	:	Cannot be used in unconscious patients
Age	:	Tablets or capsules are not suitable for neonates.

Disease status : Reduced effect in case of GI disorders
Compliance : Not effective in noncooperative patients
Rapidity : Effect produced is not very fast and it is not a preferred route in emergencies.
Accuracy : Food interactions, altered GI motility, concurrent administration of drugs, first pass effect can alter bioavailability of drug and precise concentration can not be achieved.
Adverse effects : GI side effects are very common with oral administration.

Some drugs cannot be given by oral route as they are destroyed by GI tract. Ex. Insulin, adrenaline. Enteric coated tablets resist their disintegration in stomach. Disintegration is permitted only in intestines. It reduces gastric irritation and prolongs the absorption. Controlled release preparations are designed to release specific amount of drug after specific time. These formulations offer predictable absorption of drugs.

First pass effects, enterohepatic circulation and food interactions are associated only with oral route.

Intravenous route of administration

It is a route in which drug is administered into veins. It is the only route that has 100% bioavailability because there is no concept like absorption and the drug is directly introduced into the circulation.

Advantages

i) Consciousness: IV drugs can be given to unconscious individuals.
ii) Age: This route can be used in neonates or any age
iii) Compliance: Patient participation is not required and it is an effective route in noncooperative patients
iv) Accuracy: Food interaction, concurrent administration of an other drug, first pass effects do not alter bioavailability. Hence precise amount can be administered.
v) Rapidity Action is immediate: preferred in emergencies.
vi) Adverse effects GI adverse effects can be avoided in this route: IV administration is possible in presence of GI disorders.

With IV route, one is sure that 100% administered drug is in the circulation.

Limitations

Expertise : Self administration is not possible and technical expertise is required.
Costly route : Cost of formulation, syringe, and administration.
Reversibility : Once administered; effects cannot be reversed in case of overdose.
Adverse reactions : Allergic reactions are more common with this route : deaths are reported. Drugs like aminophylline or nitroglycerine cause irritation after IV administration.

Rapid IV injections sometimes are associated with deaths.

Like above two routes, any route can be described logically and by considering the above mentioned factors. Remaining routes are not described in details; only salient features are mentioned.

Sublingual route of administration

Sublingual administration refers to keeping a tablet in buccal cavity under tongue and crushed or allowed to dissolve. Drugs are absorbed from buccal vessels. Fast action, no first pass effect, no food and drug interactions, safe use in GI disorders are the advantages while irritation and accidental swallowing are major limitations. If there are warning symptoms of overdose, tablet is thrown out. Ex. Sublingual nitroglycerine in angina pectoris, chewable ergotamine tablets in migraine.

First pass effect is avoided in sublingual route.

Rectal route of administration

Rectum offers a site for local application as well as for systemic absorption. Drugs are administered in enema or suppository form. Advantages include applicability in neonates and unconscious patients. First pass effect is partially avoided. Vomiting, upper GI disorders and food interactions do not limit rectal administration of drugs. Disadvantages include unwillingness for administration and incomplete absorption. Some more advantages and disadvantages can be derived logically by studying factors governing the routes of administration. Ex. Antibiotic suppositories for systemic administration or steroids in ulcerative colitis for local action.

Inhalational route of administration

Drugs are introduced along with inspired air in inhalational route of administration. Some times drugs act at the site of administration (in lungs) and sometimes are absorbed in circulation and act on all systems. Advantages include self administration, rapid action, no food and drug interactions, and controlled administration. Disadvantages include cost of the device, irritation of respiratory tract. Severe bronchospasm may not allow drugs to reach blood vessels. Ex. Terbutaline inhalation for local bronchodilatation. Anesthetic agents or ergotamine (in migraine) for systemic absorption.

Inhalational route is used for local or systemic effects.

Intramuscular route of administration

Drug is introduced in muscles via IM administration. Advantages and disadvantages are very much similar to IV route except for the fact that bioavailability with IM route is not 100% and effects are not as rapid as IV route. But absorption can be improved by exercise of that muscle. Exercise improves circulation in that muscle. Irritant drugs are not usually administered by this route. Muscle pain and lipotrophy are common problems with this route. Absorption with IM route every time may not be faster than oral route.

Some drugs act better by mouth than by IM injection

Subcutaneous route: With SC route, drug is administered below skin. Advantages and disadvantage very much similar to IV route except for rapid action and 100% bioavailability. Local action can be achieved by reducing absorption further. Usually irritant drugs are not given by this route. Ex. Lignocaine administered with adrenaline produces local anesthesia for longer duration. Insulin is a common drug taken by SC route. Subcutaneous space is used for placement of depot preparations of drugs like progesterone.

Subcutaneous space is used for local effects, systemic effects and placing depots.

Intradermal route of administration:

Drug is injected inside the skin. It is a very rarely used route of administration and is preferred for vaccination and sensitivity testing.

Intradermal route is used for vaccinations or sensitivity testing.

Skin as systemic route of administration: Skin can be used as local as well as systemic route of administration. Some drugs are applied on the skin and are supposed to act at that site only while some drugs are applied on the skin but they are absorbed systemically and produce effect all over the body.

1) Innuction: Rubbing of drugs on the skin facilitate penetration through skin for systemic action: Ex. Nitroglycerine ointment in angina.

2) Iontophoresis: Galvanic currents are used to facilitate transcutaneous absorption of drugs. Ex. Salicylates.

3) Jet injections. These are injections without use of needles. Drug is introduced through skin by achieving high velocity. Ex. Insulin

4) Transdermal drug delivery system (TDD System)

It is a formulation of a drug that is to be applied on the skin. It releases specific amount of drug for a long period and the drug is absorbed through skin.

It is an adhesive patch. Outer section in patch contains drug store. Drugs through porous membrane is gradually released into compartment that is in contact with skin and the drug is gradually absorbed.
Areas for application : skin of mastoid process, chest, abdomen and arm.

Transdermal drug delivery system releases fixed amount of drug and reduces number of administration.

Drugs given by transdermal delivery

Hyoscine patch	: in motion sickness
Nitroglycerine patch	: in angina pectoris
Insulin patch	: in diabetes mellitus

Advantages offered by TDD system

i) Improved compliance due to reduction in number of administrations.
ii) Prolonged and sustained effect.
iii) Accurate release of quantity.
iv) Reduced side effects.

Drug delivery systems

In fact every formulation is a drug delivery system. To overcome the limitations of standard formulations certain novel techniques are used clinically, which are termed as novel drug delivery systems. Most of which are already discussed in previous part of this section.

i) Enteric coated tablets (Refer page 61).
ii) Controlled release preparations. (Refer page 61).
iii) Depot preparations (Refer page 29).
iv) Jet injections
v) Transdermal drug delivery systems (Refer page 63).
vi) Ocuserts: Introduction of a formulation under eyelid to release specific amount of drugs. This device eliminates repeated administrations.
vii) Artificial pancreas: It is a computerised system implanted in the body. This system measures blood sugar level automatically and releases the required amount of insulin. It almost works as pancreas.
viii) Liposomal encapsulation: Drugs are incorporated into liposomes and are administered. It facilitates targeted drug delivery. Ex. Liposomal encapsulation of anticancer agents.

DEVELOPMENT AND EVALUATION OF DRUGS

Preclinical studies

Molecules that have therapeutic potential must be evaluate thoroughly before they are used in clinical practice. Initially these drugs are evaluated in animals, which is called as preclinical testing.

Objectives of animal trials

i) Screening of various molecules for their therapeutic potential.
ii) To find out efficacy.
iii) To find out safety.
iv) Investigating pharmacokinetic parameters.
v) Searching for mechanism of actions.
vi) Comparison with existing agents.

The basic aim behind all preclinical testing is judging the predictability of drugs in human beings.

Preclinical studies are conducted in different animals, with different routes and for different periods. These studies have got some limitations. Detail description of these issues is out of scope of this section. But one thing must be kept in mind that before a new product is tried in human being, several animals and several years are sacrificed in animal testing.

Clinical trials

After establishment of safety and efficacy in animals, a drug can be tested in human beings. Any drug undergoes total 4 phases of clinical trials. After first 3 phases if the drug is found safe and effective then it is allowed in the market.

Objectives of clinical trials

i) Establishing safety
ii) Evaluating efficacy
iii) Studying pharmacokinetic parameters
iv) Finding mechanism of action
v) Comparison with existing treatment.

Some techniques used to maintain reliability and ethics in studies

1) Use of control drug: Suppose a drug is found to improve some symptoms in some disease, it may not be the effect of drug. It can be the natural course of disease (e.g. Symptoms of common cold are self limiting after 2-3 days). To confirm that the improvement is due to test drug, it is compared with placebo. Some patients in the trial will receive placebo (dummy medication) while some will receive test drug. If improvement is observed only in the group receiving test drug and if the difference is statistically significant, the drug is said to be effective. Similarly test drug is compared with any standard drug that has similar type of action. Studies according to agent compared are called as placebo controlled (test drug x placebo) or positive controlled (test drug x standard treatment) studies or uncontrolled (no control).

2) Randomization: It is the random allotment of test drug or placebo to the patients. Randomization is done with the help of table of random number or computerized programmes. According to that fixed pattern patients in the trial will get either placebo or test drug. It avoids bias in the recruitment.

3) Blinding:

i) Single blind trials: If individual in the trial knows that he is receiving placebo or test drug, the psychological interpretations may alter the effect. To avoid this, patients are not informed whether they are receiving placebo or test drug. This is single blind trial. It avoids patient bias.

ii) Double blind trial: If the investigator in the trial knows what patient has received; drug or placebo, his psychological factors can alter the results. In double blind trials, neither patient nor investigator knows who is taking test medication and who is taking placebo. This design of trials avoids bias of patient and investigator.

Cross over design of trial

Suppose in a clinical trial, individuals in group A receive test drug and those in group B receive placebo, after completion of the trial there is a drug free period (wash out period) to abolish the total effect of drug. Then individuals in group A will receive placebo and those in group B will get test drug. The analysis of two steps is done together. This cross over design of the trial reduces individual variation in the trial and needs small number of patients.

Prospective and retrospective trials

When objectives of the trials are decided first and then the drug is tested it is prospective trial. In retrospective trial, first the drug is tested, data is collected and analyzed without specific objectives in mind.

Consent

Written consent must be obtained from individuals that are to be included in the trial. They must be informed about the drug administration, procedures and consequences of the drug effects. They are free to withdraw themselves from the trial at any point.

Ethics committee

Ethics committee must approve the protocol of the trial. It is formed by doctors, pharmacologists and some non-medical individuals. The committee assures ethical issues in the clinical trials.

Clinical trials are conducted in four phases: Phase 1,2,3 and 4.Drug is marketed after successful completion of phase 3 clinical trial.

Phase 1 clinical trials are conducted in healthy volunteers. The primary objectives of phase 1 studies are to find out safety and pharmacokinetic parameters of that drug in healthy individuals.

Phase 2 trials are conducted in small number of patients of the disorder for which the drug is designed. Efficacy and safety of the drug in patients is confirmed in phase 2 studies. These studies are also directed to find out mechanism of action of study drug.

Phase 3 clinical trials are conducted at various centers and in large number of patients. These studies confirm the conclusions in previous trials in large and varied population. Additionally phase 3 trials compare efficacy and safety of test drug with current standard treatment.

After successful completion of phase 3 trials drug is allowed in the market.

Phase 4 trial is also called as post-marketing surveillance. Any drug when is present in the market large number of population gets access for the drug and vast data can be collected about that drug. In these trials information about the test drug is collected from the prescribers. Personal experiences of practitioners are studied to find out new indications or side effects that are not observed in previous trials.

DRUGS IN AUTONOMIC NERVOUS SYSTEM (ANS)

"THIS SECTION CONTAINS"

Nervous system has two divisions

Central Nervous System (CNS): It includes brain and spinal cord.

Peripheral Nervous System (PNS) includes somatic and autonomic nerve fibres. Somatic Nervous System deals with voluntary functions and provide nerve supply to skeletal muscles.

Autonomic nervous system (ANS): It is the part of nervous system that deals with involuntary functions. It is also called visceral nervous system and it functions below conscious level. Pumping of heart, contraction of blood vessels, intestinal contractions, etc. are some functions that are under control of ANS.

ANS deals with involuntary functions

Anatomical formation of ANS: (Refer Figure 2.1)

Specialized areas in brain that govern ANS are not clearly defined. Hypothalamus mainly regulates autonomic functions. The next step of ANS is midbrain and spinal cord. From midbrain or spinal cord, some nerve fibres emerge and they are called preganglionic neurons. They end in autonomic ganglion where they synapse with another neuron called postganglionic neuron. Postganglionic neurons come out from ganglion and travel to different organs and end in different organs. The junction of postganglionic neuron and visceral organ is called neuroeffector junction.

Figure 2.1 Formation of ANS

Hypothalamus

↓

Spinal cord or midbrain

↓

Preganglionic fibre

↓

Autonomic ganglion

↓

Postganglionic fibre

↓

Neuroeffector junction

Heart, blood vessels, GI tract, urinary tract, respiratory tract, eye, hair follicles, spleen receive nerve supply from ANS.

Functioning of ANS: (Refer Figure 2.2)

ANS works through neurohumoral transmission. It is the transfer of message from nerve to nerve or from nerve to organs with the help of chemical messengers.

Neurohumoral transmission is a transfer of messages through chemical messengers.

Activation of ANS at the level of midbrain or spinal cord results in stimulation of preganglionic nerve. Stimulated preganglionic neuron releases transmitter I in the autonomic ganglion. Transmitter I stimulates postganglionic neuron. Stimulated postganglionic neuron releases neurotransmitter II at neuroeffector junction. Neurotransmitter II gets attached to different receptors on different organs and brings about various actions.

Figures 2.2 Functioning of ANS

Hypothalamus

↓ Overall control

Midbrain/spinal cord ← Activation of ANS

↓ Stimulation of preganglionic neuron

Release of neurotransmitter I ⟵ Autonomic ganglion

↓ Stimulation of postganglionic neuron

Release of Neurotransmitter II ⟵ Neuroeffector junction

↓

Stimulation of various receptors on various organs.

↓

Different actions

Two systems of ANS

ANS is subdivided into two systems, viz: Sympathetic nervous system and Parasympathetic nervous system. Both these systems usually function in opposite direction and maintain the balance of involuntary functions in body. Their actions are opposite but they are not equal and opposite. Domination of one of these two systems varies from organ to organ. Some sites do not have control of one of these systems. Parasympathetic system is mainly involved in conservation of energy while sympathetic system prepares body for intense activities. Parasympathetic stimulation leads to anabolism and sympathetic stimulation to catabolism.

Effects of sympathetic and parasympathetic system are not equal and opposite.

Parasympathetic system is anabolic while sympathetic is catabolic.

Formation of parasympathetic system: (Refer Figure 2.3)

Superior control over parasympathetic system is through anterior and medial part of hypothalamus. Preganglionic fibres originate from midbrain and sacral part of spinal cord. The centres of III, VIII, IX, X cranial nerve and gray matter of sacral part of spinal cord give rise to preganglionic fibres of parasympathetic system (the system is also termed as craniosacral outflow). Preganglionic fibres emerge out of mid brain and spinal cord and travel some distance and end in parasympathetic ganglia near various organs. Postganglionic fibres originate from these parasympathetic ganglia. Usually from 1 preganglionic neuron, 1 or 2 postganglionic neurons are originated. (exception is plexus: Auorbach's plexus). Post ganglionic parasympathetic neurons travel a short distance and end in neuroeffector junctions of various organs. Different organs that receive parasympathetic supply are: heart, smooth muscles (respiratory tract, GI tract, urinary tract, eye) and various glands (gastric, lacrimal, salivary, etc.). Most of the blood vessels (except of the face and neck), spleen, sweat glands, hair follicles do not receive parasympathetic supply.

Spleen, hair follicles, sweat glands and blood vessels (except face and neck) do not have parasympathetic innervation.

Figure 2.3 Formation of parasympathetic system

Anterior and medial part of hypothalamus
↓
Centres of III, VII, IX and X nerves and sacral part of spinal cord
↓
Preganglionic fibre (long)
↓
Parasympathetic ganglion (Near organs)
↓
Postganglionic fibre (short)
↓
Neuroeffector junctions.

Functioning of parasympathetic system: (Refer figure 2.6)

When parasympathetic system gets activated, preganglionic neurons are stimulated. Stimulated preganglionic neurons release Acetylcholine ACh (Neurotransmitter I) from nerve endings in parasympathetic ganglia. ACh that is released in ganglia stimulates some receptors in ganglion (N_N/M_1). This activates postganglionic neurons. Stimulated postganglionic neurons release ACh (neurotransmitter II) in neuroeffector junction of various organs. ACh in neuroeffector junction stimulates different cholinergic receptors on various organs and produces different parasympathetic actions. Immediately after the stimulation of receptors, ACh gets destroyed. Thus, ACh is the only neurotransmitter involved in parasympathetic transmission.

ACh is the only neurotransmitter in parasympathetic system.

Synthesis-storage release and destruction of ACh

Figure 2.4 Synthesis - Release - Hydrolysis of ACh

Choline + Acetyl Co.A
↓ Choline acetylase
ACh (stored in vesicles)
↓ ← Stimulation of nerves
Release of ACh
↓
Action
↓ Acetyl Choline Esterase (AChE)
Acetate and choline

For synthesis of ACh, neuronal axons take up choline from extracellular fluid. It combines with acetyl coenzyme A to produce ACh. Enzyme choline acetylase is required for this reaction. ACh thus formed in nerve endings, is stored in vesicles of preganglionic and postganglionic neurons. Stimulation of preganglionic nerve endings releases ACh in parasympathetic ganglia while stimulation of postganglionic nerves releases ACh at neuroeffector junction. ACh stimulates various receptors and produces actions. Immediately after the release, ACh is hydrolysed by acetylcholinesterase (AChE) and action is terminated.

Hydrolysis of ACh produces choline and acetate. Choline is again utilized for formation of ACh.

Pseudocholinesterase (Butyrcholinesterase): It is similar to AChE but is not present in neuronal junctions and ganglia. It predominantly present in plasma and liver. It hydrolyses ACh in the circulation. It has pharmacogenetic importance (Refer page 46).

Effects of ACh in parasympathetic system

1) ACh released by preganglionic nerve stimulates postganglionic neuron.

2) ACh released by postganglionic nerve endings stimulates cholinergic receptors on various organs.

Cholinomimetic receptors

Receptors that are stimulated by ACh are termed as cholinomimetic or cholinergic receptors. They are of 2 types- muscarinic receptors (M) and nicotinic receptors (N).

Figure 2.5 Cholinergic receptors

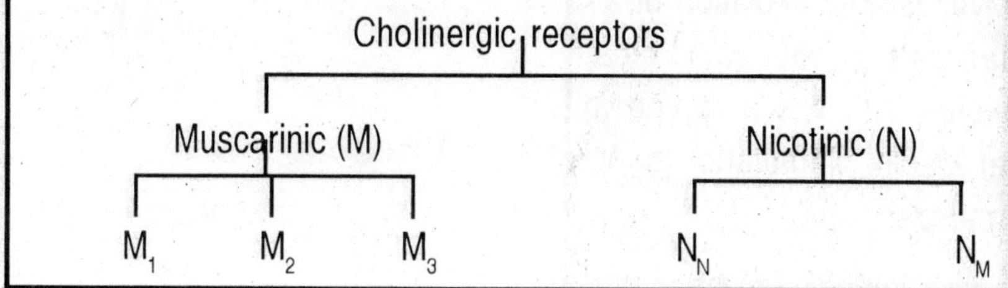

The basis for terms muscarinic and nicotinic is selectivity of these receptors. Both types of receptors are simulated by ACh but M receptors are selectively stimulated by substance muscarine and N receptors by nicotine. To understand mechanism of action of these receptors in details, brief revision of mechanisms of receptor action (Refer page 33) is essential.

All muscarinic receptors are 'G protein coupled' receptors and nicotinic receptors are 'receptors with intrinsic ion channels'.

M_1 receptors: These are G protein coupled receptors and act through IP_3/DAG mechanism by increasing cytosolic calcium in cells. (Refer page 33).

Table 2.1 Location and functions of M_1 receptors

Location of M_1 receptors	Effects
Autonomic ganglia	Weak secondary action
Nervous system	Complex undefined actions

M_2 receptors: These are G protein coupled receptors and act by opening K^+ channels or by reducing cyclic AMP. (Refer page 33).

Table 2.2 Location and functions of M_2 receptors

Location of M_2 receptors	Effects
Heart	Negative inotropic (↓ force of contraction) Negative chronotropic (↓ heart rate) Negative dromotropic (↓ conduction)

M_3 receptors: These also are G protein coupled receptors and act through IP_3/DAG mechanism by increasing cytosolic calcium.

Table 2.3 Location and functions of M_3 receptors	
Location of M_3 receptors	**Effects**
GI smooth muscles	Contraction of muscles
Bronchial smooth muscles	bronchoconstriction
Urinary tract	See below
Eye	See below
Salivary, lacrimal and gastric glands	Increased secretions

Urinary tract: Stimulation of M_3 receptors contracts detrusor (a muscle of urinary bladder) and relaxes trigone and facilitates micturition. Uteric contractions are also induced by stimulation of M_3 receptors.

Eye: (Refer figure 2.18) Iris contains two types of smooth muscles. Sphincter pupillae and dilator pupillae (radial muscles). Contraction of sphincter pupillae constricts pupil (Miosis) and contraction of radial muscles produces dilatation of pupils (Mydriasis). Stimulation of M_3 receptors contracts sphincter pupillae and produces miosis. Additionally eye contains ciliary muscles that are involved in adjustment of lens for distant and near vision. Stimulation of M_3 receptors produces contraction of ciliary muscles.

N_N receptors: These are the receptors with intrinsic ion channels. Stimulation of N_N results in opening of Na^+, K^+ and Ca^+ Channels

Table 2.4 Location and functions of N_N receptors	
Location of N_N receptors	**Effects**
Autonomic ganglia (Sympathetic and Parasympathetic)	Stimulation of postganglionic neuron
Adrenal medulla	Release of adrenaline and some noradrenaline
CNS	Complex undefined actions

N_M receptors are associated with somatic or skeletal nervous system and are present on skeletal muscles.

N_M receptors: These also are receptors with intrinsic ion channels. Stimulation of N_M receptors open Na^+ and K^+ channels. They are a part of somatic nervous system.

Table 2.5 Location and functions of N_M receptors	
Location of N_M receptor	**Effects**
Neuromuscular junction (junction of somatic nerve and skeletal muscles)	Contraction of skeletal muscles

Figure 2.6 Functioning of parasympathetic system at a glance

Superior control by anterior and medial part of hypothalamus

↓

Midbrain and sacral part of spinal cord ← Stimulation of parasympathetic system

↓

Stimulation of preganglionic neuron

↓

Release of ACh in parasympathetic ganglion

↓

Stimulation of N_N and M_1 receptors in ganglion

↓

Stimulation of postganglionic neuron → Immediate destruction of ACh by AChE

↓

Release of ACh in neuroeffector junction

↓

Stimulation of various receptors on various organs → Immediate destruction of ACh by AChE

↓

Receptors and actions

- M_1: Actions on autonomic ganglia and CNS
- M_2: ↓ heart rate; ↓ force of contraction; ↓ conduction in heart
- M_3: Contraction of all smooth muscles; Relaxation of sphincters; ↑ secretion of glands; Miosis.
- N_N: Release of adrenaline and NA from adrenal medulla.

(N_M receptors are a part of somatic system: so they are not included in this presentation)

Cholinomimetic or parasympathomimetic drugs

Drugs that stimulate parasympathetic system are called as cholinomimetic drugs.

Figure 2.7 Cholinomimetic Drugs

Cholinomimetic Drugs

- Directly acting
  - Choline esters
    - ACh
    - Methacholine
    - Carbachol
    - Bethanechol
  - Cholinomimetic alkaloids
    - Muscarine
    - Pilocarpine
- Indirectly acting
  - Anticholinesterases
    - Physostigmine
    - Neostigmine
    - Pyridostigmine
    - Edrophonium
    - Ambenonium

Cholinomimetic agents are primarily used to increase tone of smooth muscle of GIT, urinary tract and iris.

CHOLINE ESTERS

These cholinomimetic agents include ACh, methacholine, carbachol and bethanecol. These agents are rarely used in practice.

Mechanism of action: ACh and methacholine stimulates M as well as N receptors while bethanechol and carbachol have selective muscarinic actions.

Pharmacological actions:

Muscarinic actions:

i) Decreased heart rate, decreased force of contraction of heart and reduced conduction in heart. (Refer page 71).

ii) Though blood vessels do not have parasympathetic nerve supply, they contain cholinergic receptors, stimulation of which releases EDRF (endothelium dependant relaxing factor: This most probably is nitric oxide: NO). EDRF produces vasodilatation.

iii) Increased secretion of some glands: salivary, respiratory glands, lacrimal glands and increased acid secretion in stomach.

iv) Contraction of GI smooth muscles and relaxation of sphincters: facilitating defecation

v) Contraction of detrusor of bladder and relaxation of trigone-facilitating urination.

vi) Eye: Contraction of circular muscles-miosis (constriction of pupil and contraction of ciliary muscles-loss of accommodation. (Refer page 72).

vii) Bronchoconstriction.

Nicotinic action

Only ACh & methacholine have nicotinic actions. In addition to direct action they stimulate all sympathetic and parasympathetic ganglia and produce complex actions. They also release adrenaline from adrenal medulla (by their action on N_N receptors) and produce skeletal muscle contractions (by their action on N_M receptors).

Indications: ACh is not used in practice as it is immediately destroyed by AChE. Carbachol and bethanechol are not destroyed by AChE and they have selective action on GI and urinary tract. They facilitate intestinal movements (by contracting muscles and relaxing sphincters) and are used in paralytic ileus. Similar effects on urinary tract make these agents useful in urinary retention. The agents rarely are used as miotic agents.

ACh cannot be used clinically because it is immediately destroyed by AChE.

Adverse effects and contraindications: Adverse effects of choline esters usually are extensions of pharmacological actions: bradycardia, arrhythmia, hypotension, GI discomfort, breathlessness, hyperacidity. Due to these adverse effects these agents are obviously contraindicated in peptic ulcer, bronchial asthma, hyperthyroidism and hypotension.

Bethanechol and carbachol are used for urinary retention and paralytic ileus.

Individual agents

Dose: Carbachol: 1- 4 mg oral. Also available in injectable form or eye drops. Bethanechol: 10-30 mg oral TDS.

CHOLINOMIMETIC ALKALOIDS

These agents are directly acting parasympathomimetic agents and are very much similar to choline esters. They predominantly stimulate muscarinic receptors and produce actions that are similar to choline esters (Refer page 74). Ex. Muscarine, pilocarpine and arecholine

Indications: Pilocarpine is the only cholinomimetic alkaloid used in practice. It is used for its action on eye. It contracts sphincter pupillae (constricts the pupil) and also contracts ciliary muscles. Both these actions improve drainage of aqueous humor in glaucoma and reduce intraocular tension. (Refer page 103). Pilocarpine 2-4% eye drops are used in glaucoma. Pilocarpine ocusert is a depot preparation of pilocarpine for long term application.

Pilocarpine is the only cholinomimetic alkaloid clinically used.

Adverse effects of pilocarpine are rare as it is not used systemically, but sometimes ocular administration can produce systemic toxicity.

ANTICHOLINESTERASES (AntiChEs)

Introduction: These are indirectly acting parasympathomimetic agents. They inhibit acetylcholinesterase (AChE), an enzyme that is required for the destruction of ACh. Some agents of this class inhibit AChE reversibly while some irreversibly. Refer figure 2.8.

Mechanism of action

Cholinesterase (ChE) is an enzyme that destroys the ACh released from nerve endings and terminates the action of ACh. AntiChEs inhibit the enzyme cholinesterase and prevent destruction of ACh and potentiate parasympathomimetic actions of ACh. Neostigmine has additional direct action on cholinergic receptors.

Figure 2.8. Anticholinesterases

AntiChEs

- Reversible antiChEs
  - Physostigmine
  - Neostigmine
  - Pyridostigmine
  - Edrophonium
  - Ambenonium
- Irreversible antiChEs
  - OP compounds:
    - Diazinon-(TIK 20)
    - Dyflos
    - Parathion
  - Propoxur (BAYGON)

Pharmacological actions

The ultimate effect of these agents is potentiation of action of ACh, hence effects are very much similar to that of ACh or choline esters. It is like stimulation of parasympathetic system. (Refer page 74).

AntiChEs potentiate effects of ACh.

Indications

Only reversible anticholinesterases are used clinically. Irreversible agents are used as pesticides.

AntiChEs are predominantly used in GI tract, eye and neuromuscular junction disorders

i) Myasthenia gravis (Refer page 79). It is the autoimmune disease characterized by destruction of nicotinic receptors on skeletal muscles. It results in weakness and reduces capability of contraction of muscles. Anticholinesterases, by inhibiting breakdown of ACh, potentiate the action of ACh and improve contractions of skeletal muscles. Neostigmine is usually preferred.

In myasthenia gravis, in case of problems in swallowing and chewing, these agents are administered half an hour prior to meals.

ii) Glaucoma: It is the condition characterized by raised intraocular tension. (Refer page 103). Anticholinesterases contract circular muscles of iris and ciliary muscles and reduce intraocular tension.

Preferred drug: Physostigmine

iii) Physostigmine, as a miotic agent, is used alternatively with mydriatics to reduce adhesions in eye in inflammatory ocular conditions.

iv) Atonic intestines: Reduced intestinal tone after operations is improved by anticholinesterases.

v) These agents facilitate voiding of urine and are used in retention of urine.

vi) Alzheimer's disease is a loss of memory due to destruction of cholinergic neurons in brain. The destruction is compensated by antiChE induced potentiation of ACh.

Frequent monitoring of CVS, RS is essential during treatment with antiChEs.

vii) Atropine poisoning: Atropine blocks cholinergic receptors and inhibits action of ACh. AntiChEs, by potentiating action of ACh, oppose the actions of atropine in atropine overdose.

viii) Overdose of skeletal muscle relaxants: Tubocurarine like agents are administered during surgical procedures to induce muscle relaxation. In case of their overdose antiChEs potentiate contraction of muscles and reverse the paralysis.

Adverse effects: Adverse effects of these agents are all extensions of pharmacological actions. Ex: Unpredictable cardiovascular effects like bradycardia and arrhythmias, bronchospasm, laryngospasm, spasms of respiratory muscle, blurring of vision, abdominal cramps, excitement, and ataxia.

Use of AntiChEs with food may reduce nausea

Individual agents and doses	Features
Neostigmine 15-30 mg oral QID 0.5-2.5 mg IM/SC	Synthetic agent Additional direct action on cholinergic receptors. Major action is on skeletal muscles and hence is used in myasthenia gravis. Less penetration in CNS and less CNS side effects. Short duration of action.
Physostigmine 0.1 to 1% eye drops 0.5-1 mg oral or IM	Natural alkaloid. No direct action on cholinergic receptors. Major action is on eye (miosis), so preferred in glaucoma. More penetration in CNS: more CNS side effects. Longer duration of action.
Pyridostigmine 60-180 mg oral	Slow onset. Less potent. Longer duration. Less action on visceral muscles and more on skeletal muscles. Preferred in myasthenia gravis.
Edrophonium 1-10 mg IV	Short acting used for diagnosis of myasthenia gravis (Refer Page 79).

Neostigmine has got no CNS toxicity.

Status: Only reversible antiChEs are used in practice. They are used as the first line agents in myasthenia gravis.

ANTICHOLINESTERASE POISONING

It is the overdose of anticholinesterases. Chances of poisoning due to reversible antiChEs are very less but irreversible antiChEs can cause fatal poisoning. They are present in pesticides and are commonly used for suicides. Dyflos, diazinon (Tik 20) and parathion are organophosphorus (OP) compounds while propoxur (BAYGON) is a carbamate.

Atropine is an antidote for overdose of antiChEs.

Signs of poisoning: AntiChEs prevent degradation of ACh. Therefore signs of poisoning are the extension of pharmacological action of ACh. All cholinergic actions are exaggerated in this poisoning.

Skeletal muscles: Twitching, fasciculations, fatigue, paralysis
CVS: Bradycardia, hypotension
Respiratory system: bronchoconstriction, breathlessness, increased respiratory secretions.
GIT: abdominal cramps, defecation

Urinary system: voiding of urine
Eye: Pinpoint pupil due to miosis, cycloplegia
CNS: giddiness, convulsions, ataxia.

Death is usually due to paralysis of respiratory muscles, increased respiratory secretions and breathlessness.

Aims of management

i) Emergency management of symptoms,
ii) Prevention of further absorption of the poison,
iii) Blocking action of ACh,
iv) Reactivating acetylcholinesterase enzyme (AChE).

Management line

Immediate cardiopulmonary resuscitation is required if patient has bradycardia; hypotension or respiratory distress

↓

Clearing of respiratory block, patent airway, mechanical ventilation.

↓

In case of convulsions: 5-10 mg IV diazepam

↓

Patient is stabilized

↓

Fresh air

Washing skin and changing clothes (These agents are excreted through sweat and can be reabsorbed from skin.)

↓

Gastric lavage to remove unabsorbed poison

↓

Immediately start atropine 2 mg IV. Repeat doses every 15 minutes up to 100-200 mg total dose. Heart rate must be maintained above 70. Pupils must be dilated sufficiently. Dryness of mouth is watched. These are all guideline of atropine effects (Atropine blocks muscarinic receptors and prevents stimulation of these receptors by excess ACh)

↓

Next step in antiAChE poisoning is activation of enzyme cholinesterase. Pralidoxime (1 gm IV or IM) is administered 4 hourly. It reactivates the enzyme cholinesterase that is inactivated by antiChEs. Reactivated AChE destroys ACh and terminates the symptoms. This drug acts only on peripheral AChE and not in the CNS. Pralidoxime is best effective if given before 12 hours. It shows no effects if given 24 hours after the consumption of poison. The class of these enzyme reactivators is termed as oximes. The other agents in this class are Diacetylmonoxime and Obidoxime: Diacetylmonoxime acts in CNS. Obidoxime is more potent.

Management of myasthenia gravis

It is the autoimmune disorder of neurotransmission at neuromuscular junction. Thymus gland produces antibodies against nicotinic receptors of neuromuscular (NM) junction of skeletal muscles. Nicotinic receptors undergo destructive structural changes. Number of these receptors can be reduced by up to 90%. In myasthenia their life is reduced to one day. This reduces contractibility of skeletal muscles, so fatigue, muscular weakness, slowing of movements are major problems in myasthenia gravis. Myasthenia is aggravated by drugs like aminoglycosides, ciprofloxacin, phenytoin etc.

Neostigmine is a drug of choice in myasthenia gravis

Diagnostic test: 2 mg Edrophonium is administered IV. If there is no improvement in 30 minutes, 8 mg more is administered. If improvement is observed in 5 minutes, myasthenia is confirmed.

Objectives of management

i) Restoration of normal muscular function.

ii) Suppression of antibodies.

Drugs used in myasthenia gravis

i) Anticholinesterases: These agents inhibit enzyme cholinesterase and prevent degradation of ACh. This potentiates the action of ACh at NM junction and increases the contractile force of skeletal muscles.

Neostigmine is a preferred agent due to its major action on skeletal muscles. It has got less CNS side effects (15 mg oral QID or 0.5 - 2 mg SC or IM). Alternatively 60 mg pyridostigmine is used. Myasthenia is a disorder of skeletal muscles and muscarinic effects of neostigmine are not required. They can be blocked by atropine in case of severe adverse effects.

ii) Immunosuppressants like prednisolone (30-60 mg/day) or azathioprine or cyclosporine can be used to suppress autoimmune reactions.

iii) Removal of circulating antibodies can be done with plasmapheresis

iv) In refractory myasthenia, thymectomy is required to prevent production of antibodies.

v) Drugs that aggravate myasthenia should be avoided.

Anticholinergic agents (Antimuscarinic agents)

Theoretically speaking, all drugs which block actions of ACh should be called anticholinergic agents. But conventionally drugs that block only muscarinic receptors are called anticholinergics. The drugs that block N_N cholinergic receptors are called as ganglion blockers and drugs blocking N_M cholinergic receptors are called as skeletal muscle relaxants.

Term anticholinergic drug is conventionally used for drugs blocking muscarinic receptors.

Figure 2.9 Anticholinergic agents

Anticholinergic agents

- Agents blocking muscarinic receptors → (Antimuscarinics or conventional anticholinergics)
- Agents blocking N_N receptors → Ganglionic blockers
- Agents blocking N_M receptors → Skeletal muscle relaxants

Atropine and hyoscine are naturally occuring agents from conventional anticholinergics. Atropine is a belladonna alkaloid. Other semisynthetic or synthetic agents are hyoscine, pirenzepine, tropicamide, cyclopentolate, oxiphenonium, etc. Details of these are discussed at the end of this section.

Mechanism and Pharmacological actions

These agents block muscarinic receptors (M_1, M_2, M_3) reversibly and prevent ACh mediated stimulation of these receptors. Therefore all actions of these agents are opposite to that of cholinomimetic agents or opposite to stimulation of parasympathetic system.

1) CNS: Stimulation of various centres (respiratory, vasomotor, vagal, etc.) reduction in tremors and rigidity associated with parkinsonism, excitement, restlessness, drowsiness. These agents block muscarinic receptors on vestibular apparatus in inner ear and vomiting centre. By this, they produce antiemetic action (Refer page 210).

2) CVS: The effects are complex and are due to interplay of actions on vasomotor centre, vagal centre and peripheral actions. Initially there is bradycardia but then tachycardia persists. Conduction is improved and there is no major change in BP.

3) GI tract: Reduced contraction and motility of GI tract, constipation, reduced acid secretion, dry mouth due to reduced salivary secretions.

4) Respiratory tract: Bronchodilatation, reduced mucociliary clearance, reduced secretion (sometimes secretion becomes thick due to reduced water content).

5) Urinary tract: reduced tone of detrusor and increased tone of trigone. Retention of urine (Refer page 72).

6) Eye: reduced lacrimation, relaxation of sphincter pupillae (Mydriasis), loss of accommodation, absence of light reflex.

Table 2.6 Indications of anticholinergic agents

Indication	Advantages offered by these agents	Agents preferred
Bronchial asthma COPD	Bronchodilatation Relief from breathlessness	Atropine, Ipratropium
Ocular examination	Mydriasis & Cycloplegia. Facilitate ocular examination	Atropine Homatropine Tropicamide Cyclopentolate
Inflammatory conditions of eye and Ocular adhesions	Relaxation of ciliary muscles:Rest to eye Alternate use of these agents with miotics prevents adhesions	
Peptic ulcer	Reduced acid secretion	Pirenzepine Propantheline
Intestinal & renal colics, spastic constipation, dysmenorrhea	Relief from colic due to smooth muscle relaxation	Dicyclomine
Preanesthetic medication	Reduced salivary and tracheobronchial secretions Sedation Reduced vagal tone	Atropine
Bradycardia following MI	Increase in heart rate	Atropine
Motion sickness (Refer page 211).	Prevention of vomiting due to blocking of M receptors on vestibular apparatus and on vomiting centre.	Hyoscine
Parkinsonism	To adjust imbalance between dopaminergic and muscarinic transmission in CNS	Benztropine Trihexiphenidyl Biperiden
Anticholinesterase poisoning (Refer page 77).	Block muscarinic receptors and prevent action of ACh	Atropine

Therapeutic categories of anticholinergics

Preanesthetic
Atropine

Antiasthmatic
Ipratropium
Atropine

Antispasmodic
Dicyclomine
Oxyphenonium

Antisecretory
Pirenzepine
Propantheline

Mydriatic
Atropine
Tropicamide
Cyclopentolate
Homatropine

Antiemetic
Hyoscine

Side effects and toxicity

Side effects and toxicity of anticholinergics include extension of pharmacological actions like: Tachycardia, hypotension, restlessness, hallucinations, convulsions, dry mouth, blurred vision, respiratory failure, difficulty in emptying bowel and bladder, etc.

These agents are contraindicated in 1) glaucoma (as mydriasis produced by these agents causes congestion), 2) prostatic hypertrophy (they cause retention) and in 3) congestive cardiac failure with tachycardia (they increase heart rate).

Anticholinergics are contraindicated in glaucoma, prostatic hypertrophy and CCF

Treatment of overdose of anticholinergic agents:

i) Cardiopulmonary resuscitation and management of raised BP and heart rate.
ii) Gastric lavage
iii) Activated charcoal to prevent further absorption
iv) Physostigmine: 10 mg SC to promote action of ACh
v) IV Diazepam (if convulsions are present)

Features of individual anticholinergic agents are described in table 2.7.

Status: These agents are widely used in almost all conditions in which they are indicated. They are used as first line agents in antiChE poisoning, motion sickness, preanesthetic medication, ocular examination, while use as second line agents in peptic ulcer, bronchial asthma, bradycardia and parkinsonism.

Drugs acting by altering parasympathetic system.

In addition to agonists and antagonists of cholinergic receptors, various agents act by altering functions of parasympathetic system.

Hemicholinium blocks uptake of choline in nerve terminals and reduces synthesis of ACh.

Vesamicol blocks transport of choline into storage vesicles and reduces store of ACh.

Black widow spider venom causes transient release of ACh from nerve endings. It initially stimulates cholinergic receptors and then blocks them.

Botulinus toxin blocks release of ACh from nerve endings and produces anticholinergic actions.

Table 2.7 Anticholinergic agents	
Individual agents & dose	**Features**
Atropine 1% eye drop 0.6-2 mg IM/IV 0.25 to 2 mg oral Up to 200 mg in OP poisoning	Prototype agent
Atropine methonitrate	In GI disorders or asthma
Homatropine 1-2% eye drops	Less potent than atropine. Persistent mydriatic effect
Tropicamide 0.5-1% eye drops	Quick action. Short action. Unpredictable cycloplegia
Cyclopentolate 0.5-1% eye drops	Quick, potent and prolonged action. More predictable cycloplegia
Hyoscine 0.3 to 0.6 mg Oral or transdermal patch	Preferred agent for motion sickness
Dicyclomine 10 - 20 mg TDS oral	GI and renal cramps, dysmenorrhea
Ipratropium bromide 40 mcg inhalation.	Bronchodilator: Second line agent for bronchial asthma
Propantheline 15-30 mg oral QID	Reduced acid secretion and peristalsis. Second line agent in peptic ulcers. Less CNS effects.
Oxyphenonium 5-10 mg oral	Second line agent in ulcer and in hypermotility disorders
Pirenzepine 100-150 mg/day	Selectively reduces acid secretion. Preferred agent in peptic ulcer
Trihexiphenidyl Benztropine, Procyclidine Biperiden	Used in parkinsonism

SYMPATHETIC OR ADRENERGIC SYSTEM

Sympathetic system mainly contributes in intense activities, and prepares body for taking proper action in crucial situations. Stimulation of sympathetic system increases catabolic activities of the body

Anatomy and formation of sympathetic system: (Refer figure 2.10)

Superior control over sympathetic system is through posterior and lateral part of hypothalamus. Preganglionic fibres originate from spinal cord: (from segments Thoracic 1 to Lumber 3 i. e. T1 to L3). Preganglionic fibres emerge out of spinal cord and end in sympathetic autonomic ganglion. Sympathetic ganglia are present at different places.

i) Paravertebral ganglia: 22 pairs on either side of spinal cord.

ii) Prevertebral ganglia: In abdomen

iii) Terminal ganglia: Near organs like bladder, rectum

iv) Intermediate ganglia: Associated with anterior spinal route. Postganglionic fibres are originated from sympathetic ganglia. From preganglionic fibre, 20 to 100 postganglionic fibres are generated. Post ganglionic fibres travel some distance and end in neuroeffector junctions of various organs. Sympathetic system provides nerve supply to: heart, blood vessels, bronchi, GI tract, urinary tract, iris, spleen, sweat glands, adipose tissue, CNS and hair follicles.

Figure 2.10 Formation of sympathetic system

Posterior and lateral part of hypothalamus

↓

Spinal cord (segments T1 to L3)

↓

Preganglionic fibres (usually short)

↓

Sympathetic ganglion (at different places)

↓

Postganglionic fibre (usually long)

↓

Neuroeffector junction.

Functioning of sympathetic system (Refer figure 2.15)

Sympathetic system when gets activated, preganglionic neurons are stimulated. This stimulation leads to release of ACh (Neurotransmitter I) in sympathetic ganglion. ACh stimulates N_N and M_1 receptors in the ganglion which stimulates postganglionic neurons. Immediately after that ACh is destroyed by AChE. The stimulated postganglionic neurons release NA-noradrenaline or norepinephrine (Neurotransmitter II) in the neuroeffector junctions at various organs. NA stimulates various adrenergic receptors like α_1, α_2, β_1, β_2, β_3.

Thus, sympathetic system has 2 neurotransmitters one is ACh and second is NA. The synthesis, storage, release and destruction of ACh has already been discussed (Refer page 70).

Adrenergic system has two neurotransmitters. ACh in ganglia and NA at neuroeffector junction

Adrenergic receptors are of two types Alpha and Beta

SYNTHESIS-STORAGE-RELEASE-DESTRUCTION OF NA

Figure 2.11 and subsequent discussion explains synthesis-storage-release-destruction of NA.

Figure 2.11 synthesis-storage-release-destruction of NA

Tyrosine (taken up from extracellular fluid by axon)
↓← Hydroxylase
Dopa
↓ ← Dopa decarboxylase
Dopamine (in granules)
↓ ← Dopamine β oxidase
NA (stored in granules)
↓
Release of NA
↓
Stimulation of receptors - Various action of NA
↓
NA → Uptake by various mechanisms.
MAO | COMT
Intermediate → ↓ COMT → VMA → ↓ → For excretion
Normetanephrine → For excretion
Normetanephrine → ↓ MAO → VMA → For excretion

Conversion of tyrosine into Dopa is a rate-limiting step

NA is present in nerve ending at neuroeffector junctions of sympathetic system. It is synthesized in following manner. Tyrosine is taken into axon from extracellular fluid and is oxidized to dihydroxyphenylalanine (DOPA). Dopa further is decarboxylated to dopamine. Dopamine is transported to storage granules in nerve endings where with the help of β oxidase, it is converted into NA. When postganglionic sympathetic nerve is stimulated, this NA from storage granules is released in neuroeffector junctions. It stimulates various adrenergic receptors. Some adrenergic receptors (α_2) are situated on the postganglionic nerve endings. They are called as presynaptic receptors. The released NA in neuroeffector junction stimulates these presynaptic receptors. This stimulation reduces secretion of NA from nerve endings. In brief, it is the autoregulation of NA secretion. (Refer figure 2.12)

Presynaptic α_2 receptors reduce release of NA from nerve endings

Figure 2.12 Presynaptic receptors

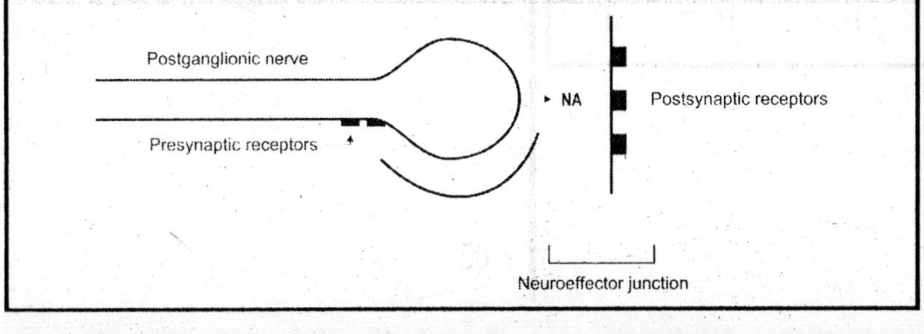

Termination of action of NA is achieved by following ways

i) Some amount of NA is taken back into nerve axons (uptake I),

ii) Some amount is picked up by postjunctional membrane (not receptors)

iii) Some amount leaves the synaptic cleft and enters in the circulation.

iv) NA is metabolised by enzymes MAO (monoamine oxidase) and COMT (catechol-o-methyl transferase) to VMA (3-methoxy-4-hydroxy mandelic acid).

The major role in terminating action is played by axonal uptake i.e. uptake of NA back into nerve (uptake 1)

Adrenaline or Epinephrine

Adrenaline is not synthesized in nerve endings but it is synthesized and released in adrenal medulla. The initial steps in synthesis of adrenaline up to formation of NA are very much similar to that of NA. Afterwards NA is converted into adrenaline by enzyme N- methyl transferase. Adrenaline is degraded by same way as that of NA.

Adrenaline is synthesized in adrenal medulla.

Figure 2.13 Synthesis-storage-release-destruction of adrenaline

Tyrosine

↓ ← Same steps as given in the figure 2.11

NA

↓ ← N methyltransferase

Adrenaline (in circulation: acts at various sites)

MAO | COMT

Intermediate Metanephrine → for excretion

↓COMT ↓MAO

VMA VMA → for excretion

↓

For excretion

Adrenergic receptors

Receptors that are stimulated by NA or adrenaline are called adrenergic receptors. They are of two types: alpha-(α) and Beta (β)

Figure 2.14 Adrenergic receptors

Adrenergic receptors

- α receptors
  - α_1
  - α_2
- β Receptors
  - β_1
  - β_2
  - β_3

α_1 receptors: These are G protein coupled receptors and act through IP_3/DAG mechanism by increasing cytosolic Ca concentration. (Refer page 33).

Table 2.8 Location and actions of α_1 receptors

Location of α_1 receptors	Actions
Blood vessels	Vasoconstriction
Iris	Contraction of radial muscles (mydriasis)
GIT	Constriction of sphincters
Urinary tract	Contraction of trigone
Glands	Increased watery secretion
Uterus	Contraction in nonpregnant uterus
Heart	Weak action
Male sex organ	Ejaculation
Skin	Contraction of pilomotor muscles.

α_2 receptors: These receptors produce their actions by various mechanisms. They alter Ca^+ or K^+ channel conduction, decrease concentration of cAMP and produce various actions.

Table 2.9 Location and actions of α_2 receptors

Location of α_2 receptors	Action
Presynaptic nerve endings	Reduced release of NA (Refer page 85)
Blood vessels	Vasoconstriction
CNS	Reduction in central sympathetic flow
Pancreas	Reduced insulin release. Increase in blood sugar levels (BSL)
Platelets	Platelet aggregation
GIT	Relaxation of GI muscles.

β_1 receptors: These are G protein coupled receptors and they act by increasing cyclic AMP concentration in the cells.

Table 2.10 Location and actions of β_1 receptors

Location of β_1	Action
Heart	Positive Inotropic (↑ force of contraction) Positive Dromotropic (↑ in conduction) Positive Chronotropic (↑ in rate of heart)
Kidney	Release of renin

β_2 receptors: These are G protein coupled receptors and they act through adenylyl cyclase by increasing concentration of cyclic AMP.

Table 2.11 Location and actions of β_2 receptors

Location of β_2 receptors	Actions
Blood vessels	Dilatation of blood vessels
Lungs	Bronchodilatation
Intestine	Relaxation
Bladder	Relaxation of detrusor
Liver & skeletal muscles	Glycogen→ Glucose (glycogenolysis) ↑ Blood sugar
Pancreas	Increased glucagon secretion ↑ BSL
Adipose tissue	Lipolysis (breakdown of fats)
Uterus	Relaxation in pregnant uterus

Role of β_3 receptors in sympathetic system is controversial and not clearly defined.

Figure 2.15 Functioning of sympathetic system at a glance

Superior control by posterior and lateral part of hypothalamus
↓
Thoracic and lumber part of spinal cord ⟵ Stimulation of sympathetic system
↓
Stimulation of preganglionic neuron
↓
Release of ACh in sympathetic ganglion
↓
Stimulation of N_N and M_1 receptors in ganglion
↓
Stimulation of postganglionic neuron
↓ ⟶ Immediate Destruction of ACh by AChE
Release of NA in neuroeffector junction
↓
Stimulation of various adrenergic receptors on various organs
↓
Sympathetic actions

Adrenergic or Sympathomimetic agents

The agents that produce actions similar to stimulation of sympathetic system are called sympathomimetic agents. Primarily they are divided as:

Figure 2.16 Sympathomimetic agents

Sympathomimetic agents

- Catecholamines ↓
  - Adrenaline
  - Noradrenaline
  - Dopamine
  - Dobutamine
  - Isoprenaline
- Non-catecholamines
  - Directly acting ↓
    - Phenylephrine
    - Phenylpropanolamine
    - Salbutamol
    - Terbutaline
    - Orciprenaline
    - Xylometazoline etc.
  - Directly + Indirectly acting ↓
    - Amphetamine
    - Tyramine
    - Ephedrine

Adrenergic system is a complex system. α and β receptors sometimes can produce opposite effects. It is the selectivity of agents for these receptors that governs final effect.

Catecholamines: The substance that contains a 'catechol' nucleus in chemical structure is called a catecholamine.

Non-catecholamines: These agents do not contain a 'catechol' nucleus in their structure.

Directly acting agents: These agents stimulate adrenergic receptors and produce actions. All catecholamines and most of the non-catecholamines act directly.

Direct + Indirect acting agents: In addition to direct action, these agents stimulate release of NA from nerve endings and produce sympathomimetic effects.

Actions of adrenergic agents vary according to their selectivity for receptors.

PHARMACOLOGY OF ADRENALINE

Adrenaline is a sympathomimetic catecholamine that is secreted by adrenal medulla.

Synthesis, release and metabolism of adrenaline is already discussed on page 86.

Mechanism of action

Adrenaline stimulates all α_1, α_2, β_1, and β_2 receptors. The net effect is the combination of the effects of stimulation of various receptors.

Pharmacological actions of adrenaline

1) **Heart:** Increase in force of contraction, rate and conduction of heart.

2) **Blood vessels:** Vasoconstriction (α_1 mediated) in cutaneous and renal vessels, and dilatation (β_2 mediated) in skeletal muscle, coronary vessels etc. The net effect is moderate rise in systolic BP.

3) **Eye:** Constriction of radial muscles of iris (mydriasis) and reduced secretion of aqueous humor. (Refer page 87).

4) **Bladder:** Contraction of trigone and relaxation of detrusor: inhibition of micturition. (Refer page 87, 88).

5) **GI tract:** Relaxation of intestinal muscles, contraction of sphincter: Inhibition of defecation.

6) **Lungs:** Bronchodilatation.

7) **Uterus:** Relaxation of pregnant uterus: Contraction of nonpregnant uterus

8) **Blood Sugar:** ↑ BSL due to ↑ in glycogenolysis, increase in glucagon and through inhibition of insulin release

9) **Adipose tissue:** Lipolysis: ↑ in free fatty acids.

Pharmacokinetics

Adrenaline is metabolised by enzymes MAO and COMT. Both the enzymes are present in GI tract. Hence, adrenaline can not be given orally. It is given by SC, inhalational, IM, IV route or applied locally. It has very short half life (2 min) and it is very short acting drug (2-3 hours). It has poor penetration into CNS.

Dose is 0.2-0.5 mg SC or IM (1:1,000 solution- 1 mg/ml IV), 0.5% inhalation.

Adrenaline is metabolised in GI tract and is not administered by oral route. It can be administered by IM, SC, IV, inhalational, local and intra-cardiac routes.

Indications

Indications of adrenaline can be remembered as: ABCDEFGH

Indications of adrenaline: A B C D E F G H

A: Anaphylaxis: (Refer page 49). It is the hypersensitivity reaction characterized by hypotension and breathlessness. Anaphylaxis is induced by histamine and adrenaline acts as physiological antagonist of histamine. Adrenaline, by increasing BP and by dilating bronchi, relieves the symptoms. It is the life saving indication of adrenaline. Additionally it acts on mast cells and reduces release of allergic mediators. It is preferably used by IM route because if used by SC route, collapsed vessels may not absorb it. IV use is dangerous.

B: Bronchial asthma: Inhalation of adrenaline produces bronchodilatation and reduces breathlessness. In severe conditions SC injections are used.

C: Cardiac arrest: Adrenaline stimulates heart and is used intravenously or by intracardiac route.

D: Dental extraction: Swab of 1:20,000 solution is applied on the site of extracted tooth. It constricts local blood vessels and reduces bleeding.

E: Epistaxis: Usually no drug treatment is required for epistaxis but local application of 1:20000 adrenaline is used in uncontrolled epistaxis.

F: For prolongation of local anesthesia (LA): Adrenaline, when is administered with LA agent, constricts blood vessels at the site and reduces the absorption of LA agent in the blood. It keeps the anesthetic agent at the site and duration of anesthesia is prolonged.

G: Glaucoma: Adrenaline mediated vasoconstriction reduces blood flow to the eye and reduces formation of aqueous humor, which in turn reduces intraocular pressure. As it causes mydriasis, it is not used in narrow angle glaucoma (Refer page 103).

H: Hypoglycemia: Adrenaline, by glycogenolysis, by increasing glucagon and by reducing insulin can increase blood sugar level.

Adverse effects

Adverse effects of adrenaline are usually extensions of pharmacological effects. Palpitations, anxiety, tremors, cardiac arrhythmia, etc. It is usually avoided in diabetes. Adrenaline is contraindicated in hypertension (as it can elevate BP), thyrotoxicosis (as it can cause tremors) and in angina (as it can increase load on heart).

Status: Adrenaline is used as the first line agent in the management of anaphylaxis. It is commonly used as second line agent in asthma and glaucoma.

NORADRENALINE

It is a catecholamine neurotransmitter of sympathetic nervous system.

Synthesis-storage-release-metabolism: (Refer page 85).

Mechanism of action:

NA predominantly acts on α_1, α_2 and β_1 receptors. It has weak action on β_2 receptors. NA predominantly produces rise in BP. Stimulation of β_1 leads to increase in force of contraction and the rate of heart which increases cardiac output (CO). Stimulation of α_1 results in vasoconstriction and peripheral resistance (PR). Increased CO and PR together increase BP (In case of adrenaline, stimulation of β_2 produces vasodilatation. Therefore, rise in BP is not as prominent as NA). Noradrenaline produces unopposed increase in peripheral resistance, due to which there is reflex parasympathetic stimulation and heart rate is reduced.

Noradrenaline produces unopposed rise in blood pressure

In clinical practice, NA is rarely used as it can cause severe rise in BP and gangrene. In extreme shocks, it is used in dose of 2-4 mcg/min by IV route.

ISOPRENALINE

It is a sympathomimetic catecholamine that selectively stimulates β receptors. It is poorly absorbed when given orally but can effectively be administered by sublingual or injectable routes.

Isoprenaline, due to its strong cardiac actions, is rarely used clinically.

Mechanism of action

Isoprenaline stimulates β_1 and β_2 receptors. It has no action on α_1 receptors. The stimulant action is more than adrenaline and noradrenaline. By stimulating β_1 receptors it increases force of contraction, conduction and rate of heart. Stimulation of β_2 leads to dilatation of blood vessels and relaxation of various smooth muscles like bronchi, intestines, bladder etc. The relaxant properties of isoprenaline can not be used clinically because of its strong action on heart.

Isoprenaline acts only on β receptors

Clinically, isoprenaline is used only in complete heart block to stimulate heart (Dose: 20 mg sublingual or 1-2 mg IM or 5-10 mcg/min IV). It is rarely administered by inhalational route.

DOPAMINE

It is a sympathomimetic catecholamine and is a precursor of NA and adrenaline. It acts through adrenergic as well as dopaminergic receptors. Additionally it is a major transmitter in CNS.

Synthesis and storage: (Refer page 85).

Mechanism of action:

It acts on α_1, β_1, D_1 and D_2 receptors

α_1 Stimulation $\rightarrow$ Vasoconstriction

β_1 Stimulation $\rightarrow$ Increased contraction, conduction and rate of heart.

Dopamine acts on D_1, D_2, α_1 & B_1 receptors and effects change according to dose.

Up to this point the action is similar to NA. Additional advantages are offered by dopaminergic action.

D_1 Stimulation $\rightarrow$ Dilatation of renal, mesenteric and cerebral blood vessels and improvement in glomerular filtration rate.

D_2 Stimulation $\rightarrow$ Reduction in release of NA from nerve endings (like α_2 stimulation)

Effects of dopamine vary with doses. With lower doses it produces dilatation of renal and cerebral vessels (D receptor mediated). Further increase in dose adds positive inotropic, chronotropic and dromotropic effects in heart (β_1 mediated). High doses produce vasoconstriction (α_1 mediated). Thus in therapeutic doses dopamine improves functioning of heart, improves blood pressure, keeping renal blood flow intact. Rise in blood pressure due to dopamine is not unopposed (like NA).

Indications

Dopamine is used to improve cardiovascular and renal function in:

Cardiogenic shock,

Septic shock and

Severe congestive heart failures are the indications for the use of dopamine (2.5 - 50 μg/kg/min IV). It can be used in combination with dobutamine.

Half life of dopamine is very short i.e. 2 minutes. It is used only when fluids in the body are sufficient.

Palpitations and nausea, are common side effects with dopamine. Marked rise in BP indicates overdose.

Marked rise in BP indicates overdose of dopamine

DOBUTAMINE

Though dobutamine is a derivative of dopamine, it does not act on dopaminergic receptors. It predominantly acts on β_1 receptors and selectively increases force of contraction of heart. It is used along with dopamine in shock and cardiac failure. Marked rise in BP indicates overdose. Dose: 2.5-10 mcg/kg/min

Dobutamine dosen't act on dopamine receptors.

EPHEDRINE

Ephedrine is a non-catecholamine sympathomimetic agent. It acts directly and indirectly. Unlike adrenaline it acts in CNS also.

Mechanism of action

It acts directly by stimulating all adrenergic receptors α_1, α_2, β_1, β_2. Through its indirect action it releases NA from nerve endings and adds to the sympathomimetic action. The actions are very much similar to adrenaline except for the fact that it acts in CNS.

Ephedrine acts directly and indirectly

Tachyphylaxis: Repeated doses of ephedrine lead to excessive release of NA from nerve endings. The storage of NA gets exhausted and fresh NA can not be synthesized with that much speed. It results in reduced effects, which is termed as tachyphylaxis.

Ephedrine produces tachyphylaxis.

Pharmacokinetics

As it is not a catecholamine, its degradation does not take place in GI tract and ephedrine can be taken orally as well as by injectable routes. It has sufficient penetration in CNS. Compared to catecholamines it acts for a longer time.

Indications

Heart block: It stimulates β_1 receptors and increases force of contraction and conduction and rate of heart.

Asthma: Stimulation of β_2 receptors by ephedrine produces bronchodilatation, hence it is used as second line bronchodilator agent in asthma.

Nasal decongestant: It contracts nasal blood vessels and reduces nasal congestion.

Ephedrine prevents ventricular systole in Stroke Adam's syndrome.

Adverse effects

Adverse effects are similar to catecholamines. Some additional CNS side effects like anxiety, restlessness and nervousness limit the clinical use of ephedrine. Dose: 15-60 mg TDS.

AMPHETAMINE

Amphetamine is a non-catecholamine sympathomimetic agent. It acts directly and indirectly. It has a predominant action in CNS.

Mechanism of action

Similar to ephedrine, through direct action, amphetamine stimulates all adrenergic receptors and through indirect action it releases NA and dopamine from sympathetic nerve endings. It predominantly acts in CNS and produces effects like; improvement in concentration and performance, postponing fatigue, improved attention, increased wakefulness, etc. Peripheral sympathetic actions are variable and unpredictable.

Amphetamine acts directly and indirectly

Indications

It is rarely used in practice as it has abuse and addiction potential due to CNS effects. Taking into account the risk involved, it can be used in:

i) Hyperactive children with attention deficit disorder,

ii) Narcolepsy,

iii) To improve sports performance,

iv) To maintain wakefulness and to postpone fatigue.

Use of amphetamine for the last two indications must be discouraged.

Dose - 5-15 mg oral BD

Use of amphetamine, except for attention deficit disorder, should be discouraged.

Adverse effects: anxiety, confusion, hallucination, tremors, GI upset, etc.

RECEPTORS AND THERAPEUTIC ADVANTAGES

Selectivity of sympathomimetic agents for different adrenergic receptors classifies them into various therapeutic categories

Agents with predominant α action on blood vessels

They are termed as Vasopressors or Decongestants.

Ex. Phenylephrine, phenylpropanolamine, metaraminol, naphazoline, xylometazoline, etc.

These agents predominantly stimulate α receptors on blood vessels and produce vasoconstriction and subsequent rise in blood pressure. These drugs are used for hypotensive emergency like shock and in arrhythmias associated with hypertension. They are contraindicated in case of thromboembolic disorders.

Sympathomimetic agents are used as decongestants

Constriction of nasal blood vessels caused by these agents relieves nasal congestion and nasal block. Most of these agents are used as nasal decongestants in anticold combinations. Depending on the individual agent, they can be applied locally or can be taken orally. Vasoconstrictor action of phenylephrine is also useful in reducing the formation of aqueous humor in glaucoma.

Agents with predominant action on β_2 receptors

They are used as bronchodilators or uterine relaxants.

Ex. salbutamol, terbutaline, salmeterol, isoxuprine, etc.

These agents predominantly stimulate β_2 receptors either on bronchi or on uterus and relax respective smooth muscles. Adrenaline though is used as a bronchodilator the action is not selective and it produces various side effects including cardiac effects. Salbutamol, terbutaline, salmeterol are the agents that have selective action on β_2 receptors and they do not produce cardiac effects. These agents are used as first line agents in management of bronchial asthma or COPD (Chronic Obstructive Pulmonary Disorders).

Salbutamol or terbutaline are used as bronchodilators.

Doses: salbutamol: 2-4 mg oral, 100 mcg inhalation, up to 0.5 mg IM. Terbutaline 5 mg oral, 250 μg inhalation, 0.25 mg SC.

These agents are also used as uterine relaxants to delay the labor or in threatened abortion or in dysmenorrhea. Vasodilator effect of isoxuprine sometimes is used in peripheral vascular disorders. Dose Isoxuprine 10-80 mg.

AGENTS WITH PREDOMINANT CNS ACTION

These sympathomimetic agents act in CNS and produce anorexiant effect by modifying release of NA and dopamine. The exact mechanism is not known. These agents make individual eat frequently but the net amount of food is reduced. Usually 15 days are required for initiation of action. Amphetamine is the prototype agent of this class but is not used clinically due to widespread peripheral effects. Fenfluramine, mazindol are similar type of agents that are preferred for the treatment of obesity. Action of fenfluramine is additionally mediated through 5HT receptors and that of mazindol through dopamine receptors. These agents are not effective for long term use. Dependence and depression after sudden withdrawal are common problems with these agents. Dose: fenfluramine 20-40 mg/day.

Mazindol and fenfluramine are used in obesity.

ADRENERGIC BLOCKING AGENTS

These agents block adrenergic receptors and produce effects that are opposite to sympathetic stimulation.

These agents are classified as:

i) α Receptor antagonists (α blockers)

ii) β Receptor antagonists (β blockers)

Few drugs block both α and β receptors

α receptor antagonists (α blockers)

These agents block α receptors and prevent their stimulation from endogenous adrenaline and noradrenaline.

Figure 2.17 α blockers

α blockers

- Nonselective
  - Non-equilibrium type
    - Phenoxybenzamine
  - Equilibrium type
    - Phentolamine
    - Tolazoline
- Miscellaneous
  - Ergotamine
  - Dihydroergotamine
  - Chlorpromazine
  - Ketanserine
  - Sildenafil
- Selective α blockers (all are equilibrium type)
  - α_1 blockers
    - Prazosin
    - Terazosin
    - Trimazosin
    - Doxazosin
  - α_2 blockers
    - Yohimbine

Nonselective α blockers: Block α_1 and α_2 receptors.

Nonselective non-equilibrium type

Phenoxybenzamine: The blockade of α_1 and α_2 receptors by it is irreversible. Any amount of NA or adrenaline does not replace the blocker from receptors.

Nonselective equilibrium type: These agents block α_1 and α_2 receptors reversibly. Excess amount of NA and adrenaline can displace these agents from α receptors.

Selective α_1 blockers: These agents block only α_1 receptors and there is no action on α_2 receptors. All of them have reversible binding with receptors.

Selective α_2 blockers: Yohimbine: It reversibly blocks only α_2 receptors and not α_1 receptors.

Miscellaneous: Agents that are listed under title miscellaneous are from different therapeutic classes, one of their property is 'α blocking' action. They are discussed in respective chapters.

Non-equilibrium type non selective α blocker (phenoxybenzamine)

Mechanism of action

It blocks α_1 and α_2 receptors irreversibly. The action is not reversed by excess secretion of NA or adrenaline.

Pharmacological actions

Stimulation of α_1 receptors in blood vessels produce vasoconstriction; hence α_1 blocking action produces opposite action, i.e. vasodilatation. Arterial dilatation causes reduction in PR and BP. Venodilatation causes reduction in venous return and postural hypotension. Stimulation of presynaptic α_2 receptors normally blocks secretion of NA from nerve endings (autoregulation: Refer page 85). Blockade of these presynaptic α_2 receptors does not block release of NA and excess NA is secreted. But α_1 on the vessels are blocked. Hence, this excess NA acts only on β_1 receptors of heart and produces tachycardia. Nasal stiffness (due to dilatation of nasal blood vessels), miosis (due to blocking of contraction of radial muscles of iris), increased tone of smooth muscle of GI and urinary tract (Due to a blocking of receptors on these muscles) are some additional effects of α blockade.

Phenoxybenzamine acts for a long time, up to 2 days and it is administered slowly (Dose: 20-60 mg/day oral or 1 mg/kg IV)

Indications: It is used only in pheochromocytoma. It is a tumor of adrenal medulla that secretes large amount of adrenaline and NA. Secretion of NA and adrenaline results in hypertension and tachycardia. Phenoxybenzamine blocks α receptors and prevents hypertensive crisis. As the binding of phenoxybenzamine to receptors is irreversible, excess adrenaline or NA can not displace it.

Irreversible blockade by phenoxybenzamine is useful in pheochromocytoma.

Side effects: These include postural hypotension (due to interference of drug in baroreceptor reflex), palpitation, nasal congestion, diarrhoea, etc.

Nonselective equilibrium type α blockers

These agents block α_1 and α_2 receptors reversibly. Ex: Phentolamine, tolazoline.

Mechanism of action, pharmacological actions and side effects are very much similar to phenoxybenzamine, except for the fact that their binding with α receptors is reversible.

The most important difference is in pharmacokinetics. These are very short acting agents and act for a few minutes.

Reversible binding of these agents limits their use in pheochromocytoma (as excess adrenaline replaces these agents from α receptors). Phentolamine is used to diagnose pheochromocytoma. 5 mg IV phentolamine over 1 minute, if reduces systolic BP by more than 35 and diastolic by > 25, it confirms pheochromocytoma.

These agents are used for short term hypertensive crisis. Phentolamine is also used to reduce dental anesthesia. Administration of phentolamine at the site of anesthesia dilates local blood vessels. The anesthetic agent is absorbed in blood and duration of action is reduced. This is required to avoid chewing of the tongue during dental anesthesia. Children or mentally retarded patients are more prone for these injuries. Phentolamine also has got direct vasodilator and cardiotonic action. Dose: Phentolamine: 5 - 10 mg IV or IM. Tolazoline: 25-75 mg oral, SC or IM. Predominant cardiac effects of tolazoline may produce rise in BP occasionally.

α_1 selective antagonists

These agents block only α_1 receptors reversibly and are most commonly used α blockers in practice.

Mechanism of action and pharmacological actions are very much similar to phenoxybenzamine. The difference is that α_2 receptors that are situated at presynaptic nerve endings are not blocked by these agents. This allows the α_2 receptors to regulate the excess secretion of NA. This reduction in NA prevents tachycardia, a major problem that is associated with nonselective agents. These drugs also inhibit enzyme phosphodiesterase. It results in accumulation of cyclic AMP. It also adds to vasodilatation.

First dose effect is sudden transient hypotension and unconsciousness after the first dose of these agents. Therefore initiation with these agents should be

First dose hypotension is common with α blockers.

Proper precaution is required while initiating therapy.

i) With minimum amount
ii) After proper information about this phenomenon
iii) Preferably before going to bed
iv) When patient is at home

Indications

i) Hypertension: These drugs are used as the second line drugs in management of HT and in combination with the first line agents. In hypertensive crisis, phentolamine or phenoxybenzamine is preferred

Selective α_1 blockers are used as second line drugs in HT.

ii) Shock: Vasoconstriction in shock is reversed by these agents. Dilatation of veins by α_1 blockers shift fluid from pulmonary circulation to systemic circulation and pulmonary edema is reduced.

iii) In Raynaud's disease and frost bite; α blockers provide symptomatic relief by improving circulation.

iv) In benign prostatic hypertrophy (BPH), α blockers relax smooth muscles of urinary tract and prostate, and improve micturition.

v) In scorpion bite, α blocker counteract sympathetic overactivity.

Side effects

First dose effect, diarrohea, dizziness and nasal congestion are some side effects of α blockers.

Table 2.12 α_1 blockers

Individual agents	Features
Prazosin 0.5 mg BD. Max: 4 mg	Prototype
Terazosin 2-10 mg OD	Long acting agent. Preferred in BPH
Indoramine 20 mg BD Max up to100 mg	Used in BPH and HT
Trimazosin 25-200 mg TDS	

α_2 Blockers: Yohimbine

It blocks presynaptic, postsynaptic and central α_2 receptors. It is a short acting agent. It is believed to be aphrodisiac (increasing sexual performance) and is used in impotence.

Sildenafil: VIAGRA: It is popularly known as a drug of decade.

Nitric oxide (NO) is the agent that is released in the blood during intercourse. This NO generates cyclic GMP which causes dilatation of penile blood vessels and maintains erection. This cGMP is degraded by enzyme phosphodiesterase 5.

Sildenafil inhibits phosphodiesterase 5 and prevents degradation of cyclic GMP and maintains erection. Side effects are mainly due to vasodilatation. They are headache, dizziness and visual disturbances. Dose 25-100 mg 1 hour before intercourse.

β receptor antagonists (β blockers)

These drugs block β receptors and prevent adrenaline and noradrenaline mediated stimulation of β receptors.

Figure 2.18 β receptor blockers

β receptor blockers

$\alpha + \beta_1 + \beta_2$ blockers	Nonselective $\beta_1 + \beta_2$ blockers	Cardioselective β_1 blockers
Labetolol	Propranolol	Atenolol
	Timolol	Metoprolol
	Sotalol	Acebutolol
	Pindolol	Butaxolol

β_2 selective blockers are of no clinical use

Mechanism of action

i) These agents block β adrenergic receptors at various sites and prevent catecholamine mediated stimulation of the receptors. Effects produced by these agents are opposite to β receptor mediated sympathomimetic actions.

ii) Intrinsic Sympathomimetic Activity (ISA). Some of the agents, along with blocking, partly stimulate β receptors. It results in moderate blocking action which can be used therapeutically. Ex: Oxprenolol, acebutolol, pindolol.

iii) Membrane stabilizing activity: β blockers, by stabilizing cell membrane, act as antiarrhythmic agents.

iv) Reduction in secretion of renin.

Agents with membrane stabilizing activity are used in arrhythmias.

Pharmacological actions

i) Heart: β_1 blockade reduces rate, force of contraction and conduction of heart. Automaticity of heart is reduced and refractory period is increased

ii) Blood vessels: Blocking of β_2 receptors prevents β_2 mediated dilatation of blood vessels and produces vasoconstriction.

iii) Bronchoconstriction.

iv) Reduction in intraocular pressure by reducing formation of aqueous humor. (Refer page 103).

v) β blockers has a minor action on GI and urinary tract

Selective β_1 blockers have got predominant action on heart.

Partial agonists or agents with ISA:

These agents have following advantages,

i) Less myocardial depression which makes these agents useful in CCF.

ii) Lesser increase in peripheral resistance.

iii) Lesser withdrawal reactions: Prolonged blockade of β receptors results in upregulation of β receptors (Refer page 33). Sudden withdrawal of these agents exposes large number of β-receptors to endogenous adrenaline and noradrenaline and sympathetic overactivity is observed. Agents with partial agonistic activity do not block receptors completely and this withdrawal reaction is not observed.

Agents with intrinsic sympathomimetic activity produce less withdrawal effects and less myocardial depression.

Pharmacokinetics

i) Propranolol follows initially first order and then zero order kinetics. (Refer page 24). Therefore their accumulation in the body is common.

ii) Propranolol undergoes first pass effect and bioavailability is reduced.

iii) Half-life of β blockers does not correlate with clinical action. Irrespective of short half life their action is prolonged.

iv) Lipid solubility: Lipid soluble agents enter into CNS and they have more first pass effect. Lipid non-soluble agents have less first pass effect, prolonged action and lesser CNS side effects. Lipid soluble agents: propranolol, metoprolol, oxprenolol. Water soluble agents: atenolol, sotalol, nadolol.

Indications

Hypertension: β blockers, by blocking β receptors, reduced stroke volume and heart rate. So they reduce cardiac output. Though their direct action on blood vessels produces vasoconstriction, after long-term use the effect vanishes. Thus, there is net reduction in BP. Additional mechanisms that help in hypertension are

i) Reduced secretion of renin: It results in reduced formation of angiotensin II which is a vasoconstrictor (Refer page 126)

ii) Reduced secretion of NA from peripheral nerve endings,

iii) Reduction in central sympathetic out flow.

Angina: Angina is the cardiovascular disorder characterized by increased demand and reduced supply of oxygen to myocardial cells. β blockers reduce HR and force of contraction of heart and reduce oxygen demand. Agents with ISA are not preferred because their partial agonistic action may not reduce heart load sufficiently.

Cardiac arrhythmias: β blockers reduce cardiac automaticity and increase refractory period. They are used in atrial flutter and fibrillations. These agents are particularly useful in arrhythmia precipitated by sympathetic overactivity.

Myocardial infarction: Immediate treatment with β blockers in MI reduces infarct size while late use prevents additional infarctions. In addition to blocking sympathetic activity, reduced platelet aggregation and enhancement of fibrinolysin probably are the advantages offered by these agents in MI. Drugs with ISA are not used in MI.

Congestive cardiac failure (CCF): Use of β blockers in CCF is controversial but these agents are found effective in mild CCF.

Anxiety: β blockers have no effects on anxiety disorder directly but these agents reduce palpitations and tremors associated with anxiety. For the same reasons these agents are used in hyperthyroidism and pheochromocytoma where there is sympathetic overactivity.

Migraine: β blockers are used for prophylaxis of migraine. As the effect is mediated through blood vessels, nonselective agents are preferred.

Nonselective β blockers are preferred in non-cardiac conditions.

Glaucoma: Timolol or betoxolol reduce intraocular tension - (Refer page 103). Compared to anticholinergic agents, β-blockers have advantage that they do not have ocular side effects: neither on pupils nor loss of accommodation.

Intraocular administration of β blockers in glaucoma does not cause loss of accommodation.

Side effects

Heart blocks, bradycardia, bronchoconstriction, sudden hypotension, sudden reduction in peripheral blood flow, interference in sleep, nightmares and sexual dysfunctions are known side effects of β blockers. Worsening of lipid profile is observed due to β blockers.

Precautions and contraindications

β blockers are contraindicated in bronchial asthma (due to bronchoconstriction) and in peripheral vascular disorders (due to peripheral vasoconstriction). During management of diabetes; understanding of warning symptoms of hypoglycemia is very crucial and these symptoms are palpitations and tremors. If β blockers are taken in diabetes, they can mask these warning signs. Additionally, hypoglycemic effects of β blockers add to hypoglycemic effects of antidiabetic agents. Body naturally corrects this hypoglycaemia by sympathomimetic mechanisms. β-blockers inhibit these mechanisms and make the situation still difficult. Use of cardioselective drugs can nullify this problem.

Cardioselective β blockers are used in presence of bronchial asthma.

β blockers are contraindicated in peripheral vascular disorders.

Cardioselective β blockers are preferred in diabetes.

Cardioselective β blockers are preferred in cardiac disorders

Table 2.13 β blockers

Individual agents	Features
Propranolol 40-160 mg/day in 2-4 doses up to 10 mg IV in arrhythmia or thyrotoxicosis	Prototype agent Lipid soluble. Nonselective. With membrane stabilizing activity. Without ISA
Atenolol 50-100 mg/day OD	Water soluble. Less protein binding. Cardioselective, Without ISA and membrane stabilizing activity. Longer half life. Preferred in arrhythmias.
Acebutolol	Cardioselective. With ISA and membrane stabilizing activity. Intermediate lipid solubility. Longer half-life
Labetolol 300-600 mg/day	Nonselective $\alpha + \beta$ blocker β blockade more potent For urgent reduction of BP Postural hypotension is common
Metoprolol 100-200 mg BD-OD	Lipid soluble, cardioselective
Timolol 0.5% eye drops	In glaucoma
Betaxolol 0.5% eye drops	In glaucoma.

Status: These are commonly used first line agents in various disorders. Usually they are used in combinations with different drugs in different disorders:

HT	:	With diuretics or calcium channel blockers, etc.
Angina	:	With nitrates or calcium channel blockers
Anxiety	:	With antianxiety agents
Thyrotoxicosis	:	With antithyroids.

In cardiac conditions cardioselective agents are preferred otherwise nonselective agents are used.

Drugs that alter sympathetic system

In addition to agonist and antagonists, various drugs produce their effects by altering sympathetic system.

α **methyl tyrosine** inhibits enzyme tyrosine hydroxylase and reduces formation of NA.

Imipramine and cocaine block uptake of NA from nerve ending and facilitate accumulation of NA at receptors.

Amphetamine and tyramine displace NA from nerve endings and produce sympathomimetic actions.

Bretylium and guanethidine prevent release of NA from nerve ending.

Management of glaucoma

Physiological considerations

Figure 2.18 Eye

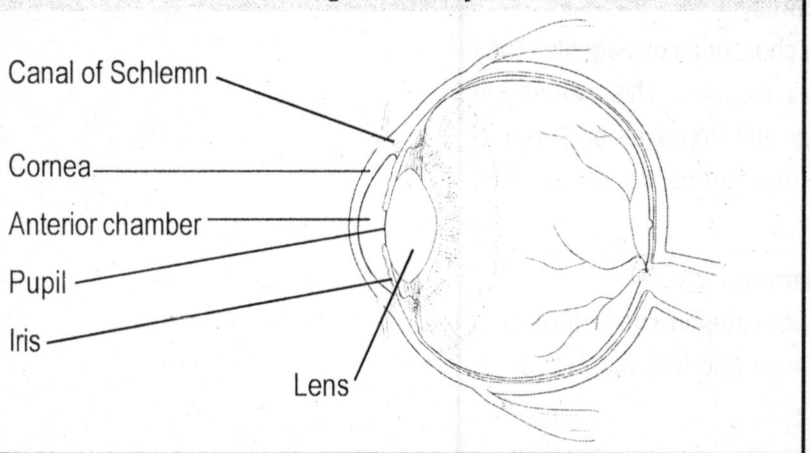

Anterior chamber of eye is formed in front by cornea and posteriorly by lens and iris. The chamber is filled with a fluid, aqueous humor. Ciliary processes secrete aqueous humor in anterior chamber, where it circulates and is drained out through trabecular network into canal of Schlem. Canal of Schelm drains it into aqueous vein. Aqueous humor maintains intraocular tension (IOT) constant (12-20 mm Hg).

Glaucoma is raised intraocular tension

Glaucoma

Glaucoma is a disorder characterized by raised intraocular tension (more than 20. It can go up to 40-50 mm of Hg). Glaucoma produces pain in eye and can damage optic nerve and cause blindness. Glaucoma is of two types.

i) Narrow angle or congestive glaucoma: In this type of glaucoma, angle between iris and cornea becomes narrow and canal of schlem is obliterated. This blocks the drainage of aqueous humor and IOT is raised.

ii) Wide angle glaucoma: In this type of glaucoma, the angle is normal. But due to degenerative changes in trabeculae, drainage system of aqueous humor is affected.

Objectives of management

1) Reducing IOT to reduce pain and to prevent damage of optic nerve,
2) Improving drainage of aqueous humor, and
3) Reducing formation of aqueous humor.

Miosis reduces pain in congestive glaucoma.

Figure 2.20 Drugs used in management of glaucoma

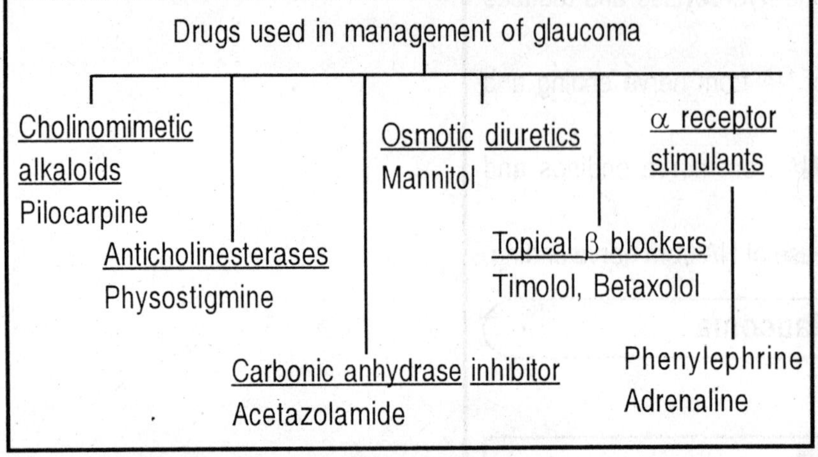

Mechanism by which drugs act in glaucoma

i) Pilocarpine and physostigmine: They are cholinomimetic agents. They contract circular muscles of iris and ciliary muscles. This widens the obliterated angle between iris and cornea and improves drainage of aqueous humor. Dose: Pilocarpine 2% eye drops or ocusert and physostigmine 0.5% eye drops.

ii) Carbonic anhydrase inhibitor: Acetazolamide.
Acetazolamide reduces availability of bicarbonates in eye and prevent formation of aqueous humor. (Acetazolamide 250-500 mg oral or IV. OD-BD).

iii) Osmotic diuretics -mannitol:
This is an osmotically active substance. It increases transport of fluids from aqueous humor into blood, which reduces the volume of aqueous humor and pressure in anterior chamber. It is used only in severe cases and by IV route in dose of 20 mg.

iv) Topical β blockers: Recently, β blockers are used as drugs of choice in glaucoma. These agents probably reduce formation of aqueous humor and provide relief. Ocular adverse effects like loss of accommodation, absence of light reflex and miosis are not present with these agents. These effects are commonly observed with pilocarpine or physostigmine. Betaxolol has selective ocular action (0.5% eye drops) Timolol 0.5% drops

β blockers, in glaucoma, provide relief without ocular side effects like loss of accommodation and impaired reflex.

v) Alpha adrenergic agonists: These agents contract ocular blood vessels and reduce blood flow to eye which in turn reduces formation of aqueous humor and IOT. By direct action on iris muscles, these agents produce weak mydriatic action. Mydriasis leads to obliteration of the angle of eye. Hence, they are contraindicated in narrow angle glaucoma. Dose: Adrenaline 0.25 to 2% eye drops.

Alpha stimulating agents cause mydriasis and are contraindicated in narrow angle glaucoma.

Management line

Wide angle glaucoma: It is not a medical emergency and long term management is required. Topical β blockers are the preferred agents. Alternatively, pilocarpine or pilocarpine + physostigmine is used. Acetazolamide is used for long term management. α stimulants are used in refractory cases.

Close angle (narrow angle) glaucoma or congestive glaucoma

This is a medical emergency. If not treated promptly, can lead to blindness. Immediate administration of topical β blockers in combinations with pilocarpine every 10 minutes is the first line of management for better control. Acetazolamide is used for long term management. α receptor stimulants are contraindicated in this type of glaucoma. Surgery may be required if patients are not controlled on drug therapy.

DRUGS ACTING ON GANGLION

As the name suggests, these drugs act on autonomic ganglia. They either stimulate the ganglia or inhibit them. Ganglia of both sympathetic and parasympathetic system are the same. (i.e. the mediator is common-ACh and major receptor is also common N_N) If a drug has ganglion stimulating action, both sympathetic and parasympathetic systems get stimulated, and if drug has inhibitory action, there is inhibition of both sympathetic and parasympathetic systems. Therefore effects are nonselective and unpredictable. That is the reason why these drugs are not used commonly in clinical practice.

To predict the effects of ganglion stimulants or blockers, it is essential to know which system (sympathetic or parasympathetic) has dominance at the specific site. Except for blood vessels and sweat glands; in all sites parasympathetic system is predominant.

Except for blood vessels and sweat glands: in all other organs parasympathetic system is predominant.

Parasympathetic predominance is found in heart, iris, ciliary muscle, GI tract muscles, respiratory muscles, urinary tract muscles, various glands (except sweat glands).

Secretion of sweat and control of blood vessels are under sympathetic dominance.

Male sexual function has equal control by both the systems.

Ganglionic stimulants

Drugs like nicotine, ACh, anticholinesterases stimulate autonomic ganglia and subsequently stimulate postganglionic fibres of sympathetic and parasympathetic systems.

Drugs acting on ganglion are rarely used in clinical practice due to their widespread actions.

Figure 2.21 Ganglionic stimulation

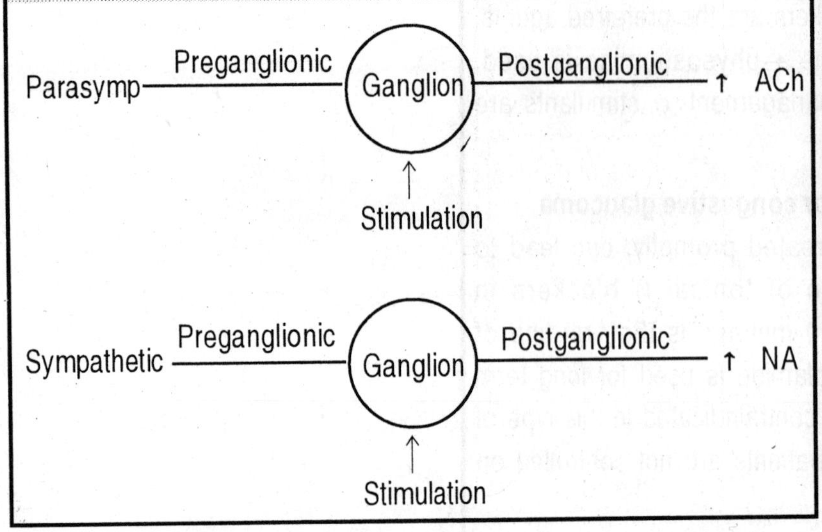

Thus ganglionic stimulants increase secretions of ACh and NA. Their effects on the body are discussed in table 2.14

Ganglion blocking agents

These agents block mainly nicotinic receptors, either competitively or persistently. Hexamethonium, Trimethophan, Pentolinium are competitive blockers. Drugs which stimulate ganglion in high doses block the ganglia persistently. Nicotine or anticholinesterases, in high doses, are persistent ganglion blockers.

Figure 2.22 Ganglionic inhibitions

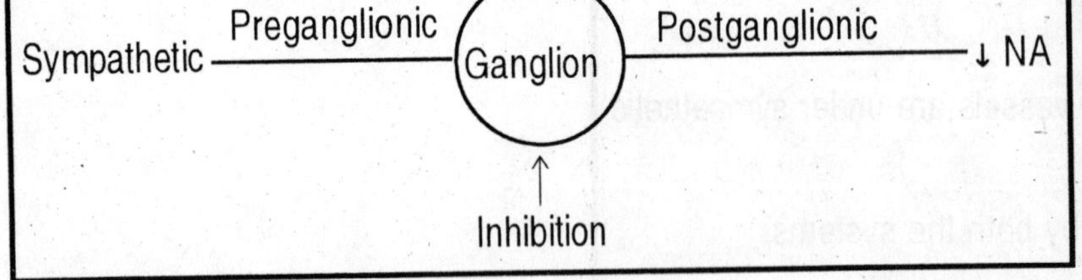

Thus ganglionic blockers inhibit release of ACh and NA but the net effects again depend upon predominance. Their effects on the body are discussed in table 2.14

Indications: Nonselectivity and unpredictability of these agents limit their use in clinical practice. Trimethophan is occasionally used in hypertension.

Table 2.14 Effects of drugs on autonomic ganglia			
Site	**Predominant system**	**Effect of ganglionic stimulants**	**Effect of ganglionic blockers**
Heart	PS	↓ HR, ↓ force of contraction ↓ conduction	Tachycardia Palpitation
GIT	PS	↑ Contractibility ↑ Secretions	↓ Motility ↓ Secretions Constipation
Respiratory tract	PS	Bronchoconstriction ↑ Secretions	Bronchodilatation ↓ Secretions
Eye	PS	Miosis, Loss of accommodation	Mydriasis, Loss of accommodation
Urinary tract	PS	↑ tone of detrusor muscle. Relaxation of sphincters. Voiding of urine	Opposite effects Difficulty in micturition
Glands	PS	↑ Salivation ↑ Lacrimation	Dry mouth Dry eyes
Male Sexual function	PS symp	Stimulation of erection and ejaculation	Inhibition of ejaculation and erection
Blood vessels	symp	Vasoconstriction ↑ PR, ↑ BP	Vasodilatation ↓ PR, ↓ BP
Sweat Glands	symp	↑ Sweating	Reduced sweating

PS: Parasympathetic system
Symp: Sympathetic system.

NICOTINE

Nicotine, though stimulates autonomic ganglia, in large doses produces persistent depolarization and block ganglia. The net pharmacological actions are as follows.

CNS: Stimulation of CNS, tremors, convulsions with large doses, vomiting due to stimulation of CTZ (Chemoreceptor Trigger Zone), dependence.

Adrenal medulla: Release of adrenaline, sympathetic stimulation, increase in heart rate and PR.

Skeletal muscles: twitching

Metabolic effects: ↑ Basal Metabolic Rate, Hepatic microsomal enzyme induction, lipolysis, etc.

Consequences of chronic smoking or chewing tobacco:

i) Lung carcinoma: due to carcinogenic potential

ii) Chronic obstructive pulmonary disorders: due to irritants in smoke,

iii) Oral malignancies: due to carcinogenic potential of tobacco. Tobacco chewing is predominantly associated with oral malignancies.

iv) Ischemic heart diseases: Sympathetic overactivity by nicotine results in a) Increased contractibility of heart b) Increased PR c) Altered lipid profile d) Increased platelet aggregation.

v) Peripheral vascular disorders: reasons same as above.

vi) Acid-peptic disorders: due to excess acid secretion by nicotine.

Treatment for tobacco dependence

i) Gradual withdrawal

ii) Psychotherapy

iii) Transdermal nicotine patches.

AFFERENT COMPONENT OF ANS

Baroreceptor reflex: Though ANS is predominantly involved in efferent activities, it has got important afferent network. The classical example is baroreceptor reflex.

Mechanism of baroreceptor reflex

Increased blood pressure

↓

Stimulation of sensory receptors in aortic arch and carotid sinus

↓

Message to vasomotor centre

↓

Inhibition of sympathetic system or activation of parasympathetic system

↓

Reduced heart rate and peripheral vasodilatation.

↓

Reduced blood pressure

Similarly reduction in blood pressure through reflex activity produces rise in blood pressure. Drugs that reduce blood pressure may activate this reflex and their effect is modified. Ex: Some antihypertensives cause sudden drop in blood pressure, which reflexly stimulates sympathetic system and produces opposite effect, i.e.rise in BP.

Reflex stimulation of ANS can modify effects of drugs

SKELETAL MUSCLE RELAXANTS

Physiological considerations

Skeletal muscles are under voluntary control and somatic nervous system is involved in contraction of these muscles. Somatic nerves are initiated in the spinal cord and directly end-up in skeletal muscles forming neuromuscular junction (NM junction). There are no ganglia involved in this system. ACh is the only neurotransmitter that is released at NM junction. It gets attached to N_M receptors and stimulates them which results in contraction of muscles.

Somatic nerves do not have ganglia.

Skeletal muscle relaxants

These agents reduce tone of skeletal muscle. They are classified as:

Figure 2.23 Skeletal muscle relaxants

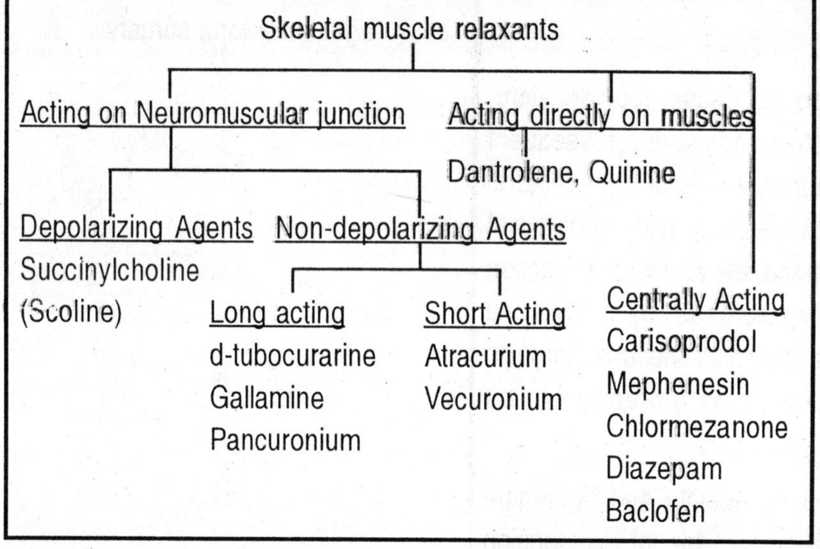

Neuromuscular blocking agents are used only after induction of anesthesia.

DEPOLARIZING AGENTS

The classical agent in this class is suxamethonium (scoline). It is structurally similar to ACh. It acts on neuromuscular junction and produces skeletal muscle relaxation.

Mechanism of action: In NM junction (of skeletal muscles), scoline gets attached to N_M receptors and initially stimulates the receptor. It is not destroyed by enzyme cholinesterase and action is not terminated. ACh in NM junction can not displace the drug from the receptors. The continued depolarization of muscle cells due to drug initially produces contractions- fasciculations and then permanent depolarization that leads to relaxation. After this, it acts like non-depolarizing competitive agent. (see below). Then it is destroyed in body by pseudocholinesterase (Refer page 71). Administration of neostigmine (anticholinesterase) inhibits pseudocholinesterase and prevents inhibition of the scoline and potentiates muscle relaxation. Genetic deficiency of pseudocholinesterase exaggerates the action of scoline and results in paralysis of respiratory skeletal muscles: scoline apnea. Action of scoline starts within a minute and lasts for around 4 minutes. It is used mainly for short surgical procedures. Dose: 1 mg/kg to start with and then as per the requirement.

Adverse effects: Bradycardia, extrasystole, cardiac arrest, premature labor and post operative pain are side effects with scoline. Scoline apnea (see above) and malignant hyperthermia are serious side effects of scoline. The drug should be given with caution in skeletal muscle and collagen disorders.

NON-DEPOLARIZING AGENTS

These include d-tubocurarine, gallamine, pancuronium etc. They act on NM junction but the mode of action is different from that of depolarizing agents.

Scoline is used for short surgical procedures while d-tubocurarine like agents for long surgery.

Mechanism of action

These agents occupy N_M receptors but do not cause depolarization. They inhibit attachment of ACh to N_M receptors and prevent subsequent stimulation of receptors. In a way they are antagonists of N_M receptors. The antagonism is reversible. If amount of ACh is increased in NM junctions. ACh replaces these agents from the site and relaxant action is reversed. Administration of anticholinesterases, by preventing destruction of ACh, reverses the relaxant action of these agents. (In case of depolarizing agents the action is potentiated by anticholinesterases)

These agents have some ganglion blocking activity and histamine releasing potential. Both these actions are responsible for hypotension and bronchospasm, which are the common side effects. Additional side effects are respiratory paralysis, hypoxia, regurgitation of gastric juice, etc. The drug must be given with caution in respiratory acidosis or alkalosis and in myasthenia gravis.

Maximum effects of d-tubocurarine is achieved in 4 minutes and action lasts for about half an hour. The reason for termination of action is redistribution of the drug.

Individual agents from this class are described in table 2.15

Indications

1) In general anesthesia (GA): Surgeries and short procedures demand skeletal muscle relaxation. If it is to be achieved by anesthetic agents, more depth of anesthesia is required, which obviously increases the risks associated with GA. By the use of skeletal muscle relaxants that much depth of anesthesia is not required and risks are reduced. For short procedures or endotracheal intubation scoline is used while for longer procedures d-tubocurarine is preferred. Atracurium is used for short procedures. These drugs are administered only after induction of anesthesia.

2) Electroconvulsive therapy (ECT): Skeletal muscle relaxants are used while giving ECT to avoid convulsions and trauma.

3) Status epilepticus, tetanus, poisoning by convulsant substances: In all these situations, these agents are used to prevent forceful contractions of muscles.

Table 2.15 Non-depolarizing agents

Individual agents and dose	Features
d-tubocurarine 0.2-0.4 mg/kg IV	Prototype agent
Gallamine 1-1.5 mg/kg IV	Faster onset of action. No histamine release and so no bronchospasm and hypotension.
Pancuronium 0.04-0.6 mg/kg IV	More potent. Longer duration. No ganglion blocking activity. No histamine release. It has cardiac stimulatory action: hence preferred in shock
Atracurium 0.3-0.6 mg/kg IV	Short acting agent Spontaneously inactivated in body by chemical process and its action does not depend on metabolism by liver or excretion by kidney. Hence, it is a preferred agent in hepatic or renal disorders.
Vecuronium or Mivacurium.	These are ultrashort acting agents.

Drugs acting on NM junctions are used only after induction of anesthesia.

Directly acting muscle relaxant: Dantrolene

Dantrolene directly acts on skeletal muscles. It reduces release of Ca from sarcoplasmic reticulum and prevents contraction of muscles.

Indications

i) Malignant hyperthermia: It is the condition characterized by continuous release of Ca from sarcoplasmic reticulum. It results in contractions and hypermetabolic state. Dantrolene (1 mg/kg IV) is a drug of choice of this condition.

ii) Spastic muscle: 25-100 mg

Dantrolene is used in malignant hyperthermia.

Side effects: Weakness, sedation, diarrhoea, hepatic toxicity caused by dantrolene limit the use of this drug as a muscle relaxant.

Centrally acting muscle relaxants

These agents neither act on muscles nor at the junction. They depress spinal and supraspinal polysynaptic reflexes that regulate skeletal muscle tone. Benzodiazepines and baclofen are drugs that have action in CNS that is mediated by GABA receptors.

Individual agents

Carisoprodol	-	350 mg TDS
Chlorzoxazone	-	250 mg TDS
Chlormezanone	-	100 mg TDS
Methocarbamol	-	500 mg TDS (oral or IV)
Diazepam	-	5-10 mg TDS oral or IV
Baclofen	-	10-25 mg TDS

Indications

Most of these agents are used in fixed dose combinations with analgesic agents in following conditions:

i) Sports injuries: Sprains, strains, dislocations, fractures

ii) Acute muscular spasms,

iii) Rheumatic muscular pain

iv) Lumbago, backache,

v) Spastic disorders,

vi) In tetanus IV methocarbamol is used.

Side effects: Sedation, drowsiness, confusion etc.

Centrally acting muscle relaxants are used in combination with analgesic-antiinflammatory agents.

Local anesthetics (LA)

These agents, after local application or injection, produce loss of sensation (especially pain) without altering consciousness. They are commonly used for small surgical procedures or painful conditions.

Mechanism of action

LAs act on voltage gated ion channels of nerve cells. They prevent entry of sodium into cells and inhibit generation of action potential, which in turn prevents generation and conduction of impulses. LAs act on motor as well as sensory nerves. Small and nonmyelinated fibres are more sensitive for the action of LAs. Pain is the first sensation that is lost. Temperature, touch, deep pressure sensations are lost gradually. Motor fibres are less sensitive for LAs.

Absorption of LAs from the site into blood terminates the local action and induces systemic effects. The common systemic effects are euphoria, excitement, twitching, tremors, convulsions, respiratory depression, etc. Cardiovascular effects of LAs are reduced contractibility and conduction of heart. LAs have quinidine like antiarrhythmic effects when administered systemically.

Administration of LAs with vasoconstrictors

Anesthetic action of LAs is terminated by its absorption from the site of administration. If the absorption is delayed, duration of action is prolonged. Administration of vasoconstrictors along with LAs reduces blood flow at the site of administration. It reduces absorption of LAs and LAs remain at the site for a long time and action is prolonged. Decrease in absorption also results in reduced systemic side effects of LAs. But this co-administration is associated with increased local pain and necrosis at the site of injection. Vasoconstrictors are not used for LAs at extremities like finger tip or penis as vasoconstriction can result in total cutting off of blood supply to that area.

Absorption of LAs in blood terminates their local action

Pharmacokinetics

Early initiation and prolonged duration are the crucial pharmacokinetic issues with LAs. The duration is governed by blood flow to the site. LAs penetrate intact skin poorly, absorption is faster in mucosa and injured areas but very slow in inflammed area. Different agents have different onset and duration of action but usually the effect starts within 5 minutes and is maintained for 1-1.5 hrs.

Absorption of LAs is slow in inflammed areas

Adverse effects

Local effects: Pain and necrosis at the site of injection.

Systemic effects: bradycardia, hypotension, nervousness, tremors, convulsions, hypersensitivity, etc.

Individual agents: LAs are broadly divided in two types

Table 2.16 Local anesthetic agents

Types of LAs

Esters	Amides
Cocaine	Lignocaine
Procaine	Bupivacaine
Tetracaine	Dibucaine
Benzocaine	Prilocaine

Amides are preferred agents as they are more potent, longer acting and with lesser allergic reactions.

> Amide local anesthetics are more potent, longer acting and with lesser allergic reactions.

LAs, depending on their therapeutic applications, are classified as:

Table 2.17 Applications of LAs

Applications of LAs

Used only for topical applications	Used only for injectable applications	Used for both topical and injectable applications
Cocaine	Procaine	Lignocaine
Benzocaine	Prilocaine	Tetracaine.
	Bupivacaine	
	Dibucaine	

> Lignocaine is most commonly used local anesthetic agent.

Techniques used for local anesthesia

Surface anesthesia

Application of anesthetic agent on skin or mucus membrane is termed as surface anesthesia .Mucus membranes of nose, mouth, throat, pharynx, urethra are common mucosal sites for LAs. LAs are applied for surface anesthesia in various formulations like creams, suspensions, ointments, sprays, suppositories, etc.

Table 2.18 Indications for surface anesthesia

Indications for surface anesthesia

Mucus membrane: Disorders	Mucus membrane: Procedures	Skin: Disorders	Skin: Procedures
Stomatitis	Tonsillectomy	Ulcers	IV cannulation
Gastritis	Catheterization	Burns	Skin surgery
Esophagitis	Proctoscopy	Scorpion bite	
Soar throat			
Fissures			
Piles			
Ocular Irritation			

Infiltration: It is the administration of anesthetic agent under the skin to block pain sensation. With infiltration, small anesthetized area is made available for procedures like incision or excision

Lignocaine, bupivacaine or procaine is used for infiltration.

Nerve block: Anesthetic agent is administered in nerve plexuses to anesthetize a specific region that gets supply from that plexus. Ex. Brachial plexus, paravertebral plexus, paracervical plexus, lingual block, sciatic block, etc. This technique is used for short procedures, fracture reductions, tooth extraction, etc.

Field block: Field block means administration of LAs in such a way that the whole nerve supply of specific area is blocked and a large area is anesthetized. Ex. operations of upper or lower extremities or appendicectomy.

Spinal anesthesia

(Subarachinoid or intrathecal anesthesia).

Anesthetic agent is injected in subarachinoid space in intervertebral regions. (Between L-2/3 or L-3/4). The agent acts on the nerve roots in cauda equina and produces anesthesia in lower abdomen and lower limbs. The level of effect and duration of anesthesia is affected by (i) individual agent (ii) posture of the patient. Specific gravity of agent and tilting of patient can change anesthetic level. Lignocaine and bupivacaine are preferred agents for spinal anesthesia. The average duration of spinal anesthesia is 1-3 hours. Addition of adrenaline prolongs the duration

Spinal and epidural anesthesia reduce risks associated with general anesthesia.

Advantages of spinal anesthesia: Spinal anesthesia is an effective alternative for general anesthesia. It avoids cardiac and respiratory depression associated with GA. All risks of GA are eliminated by spinal anesthesia. Spinal anesthesia also provides muscle relaxation.

Disadvantages

i) Headache due to leakage of CSF from site of injection

ii) Infection at the site of injection can lead to meningitis

iii) Hypotension due to sympathetic blockade.

iv) Nausea, vomiting

Spinal anesthesia is not used in hypotension and children.

Indications

Techniques of spinal anesthesia are commonly used in pelvic and lower abdominal surgeries, lower limb fractures, obstetric procedures including cesarian. Lignocaine and bupivacaine are preferred agents.

Epidural anesthesia: (Extradural anesthesia)

Anesthetic agent is injected in extradural space of spinal cord. It acts on the roots of spinal nerves of thoracic, lumbar or sacral region. All advantages of spinal anesthesia are there with epidural anesthesia. Additionally, CSF leakage is prevented and chances of hypotension are less. Lignocaine and bupivacaine are preferred agents.

Intravenous anesthesia

It is the administration of local anesthetic agent in occluded veins of limbs. Limbs are elevated first. Then a tourniquet is applied to the limb and LA is injected in the part of vein that is distal to the tourniquet. The agent gets infiltrated in the surrounding tissues and anesthetic field is achieved. With this technique anesthesia is maintained for around 45 minutes. It is not a very safe technique and rarely used for orthopedic procedures.

Agent: Prilocaine and lignocaine.

Individual local anesthetic agents are discussed in table 2.19

LAs are differentiated by their onset and duration of action.

Table 2.19 Local anesthetic agents

Individual agents and dose	Features
Lignocaine (lidocaine) Surface - 2- 4% Infiltration 0.15-0.5% Nerve block 1% Spinal 5%	Amide agent Drug of choice for surface and injectable anesthesia. Rapid onset (3minutes). Duration upto 2 hours Less allergic reactions Used in various procedures and techniques. Also used in arrhythmias. Convulsions and psychotic reactions are common problems.
Bupivacaine 0.25 to 0.5 % for injectable techniques	Amide local anesthetic agent. Used only for injectable purpose. More potent than lignocaine. Onset within 5 minutes but peak action takes 30 minutes. Action can last upto 6hrs. Cardiotoxicity, drowsiness and convulsions are common problems.
Dibucaine 0.25-0.5%	Amide anesthetic for injectable purpose. Most potent. Most toxic. Longest duration. For long term spinal anesthetics.
EMLA: Eutectic mixture of lidocaine and prilocaine	Cream applied on skin under occlusive dressing for 1hour. It is penetrated in the skin and deeper anesthesia is produced without injection.
Procaine	Rarely used as anesthetic agent. Combined with penicillin to reduce absorption of penicilln and to prolong the duration of its action. Predominat CNS toxicity.

AUTACOIDS AND RELATED DRUGS

"THIS SECTION CONTAINS"

Autacoids

(Autos: self, akos: healing)

Autacoids are substances that have following criteria.

Production by a variety of cells in the body,

Local action at the site of production,

Involvement in various physiological and pathological processes.

Classification of autacoids: Autacoids are rarely used for therapeutic purpose but modifications in the actions of autacoids offer various advantages in clinical practice. Nonsteroidal antiinflammatory drugs (NSAIDs), Angiotensin converting enzyme inhibitors (ACE inhibitors), antihistaminics, etc. are very commonly used agents that act by modifying actions of autacoids.

Autacoids can be classified as:

Figure 3.1 Autacoids

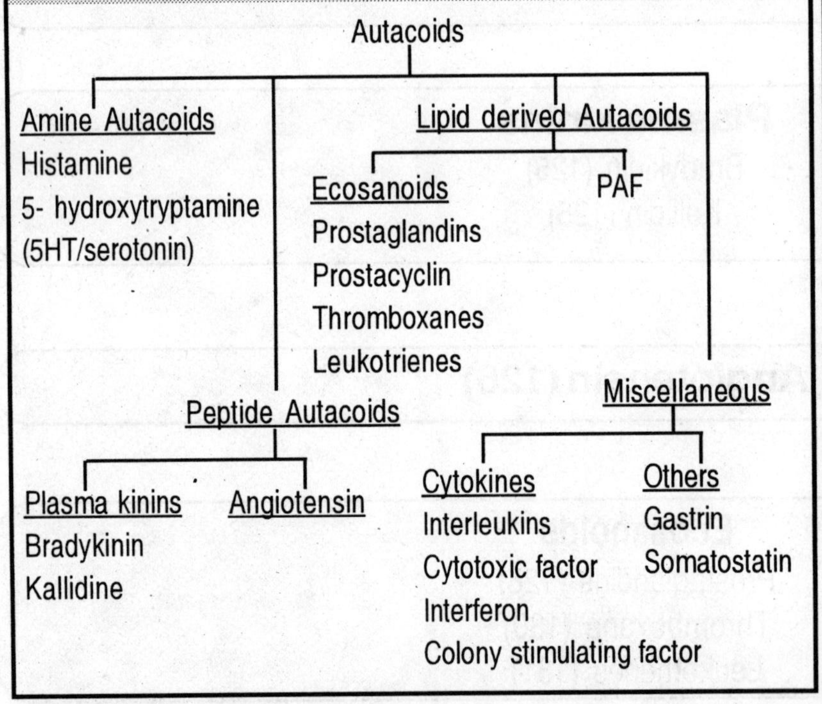

Histamine (Histos: tissue and amine type of autacoid)

This is an amine autacoid that is produced by almost all cells in human body. It is predominantly present in mast and blood cells. Skin, gastric mucosa, lungs, liver, placenta, body secretions contain histamine. It is involved in various physiological and pathological processes. Antihistaminic drugs produce their effects by blocking action of this autacoid. Histamine is not therapeutically used.

Synthesis and release

Histamine is produced from amino acid histidine in following manner. (Refer figure 3.2)

Figure 3.2 Synthesis and release of histamine

Histidine
↓ Decarboxylase
Histamine
↓
Stored in mast cell granules in inactive form (bound form)
↓
Stimuli like foreign body invasion, antigen-antibody reactions, injury, chemicals, some enzymes release active histamine in blood
↓
Histamine gets attached to Histamine 1 (H_1) receptors and Histamine 2 (H_2) receptors.
↓
Stimulation of receptors. Both these are G protein coupled receptors and their action is governed through IP_3/DAG or adenylyl cyclase mechanism
↓
Various actions. Immediate degradation of histamine takes place by oxidation or methylation

Actions and roles of histamine through H_1 receptors

1) Action of histamine on blood vessels: Histamine induces release of EDRF (endothelium dependant relaxing factor) and dilates blood vessels. This action is observed in all types of vessels. It also increases permeability of blood vessels and causes exudation of fluids and edema. There may be a fall in BP and reflex increase in heart rate. Vasodilatation of cerebral blood vessels produces throbbing headache or increase in CSF pressure.

Histamine is a mediator in bronchial asthma, allergic responses and anaphylactic reactions.

2) Histamine stimulates H_1 receptors in the lungs and produces bronchoconstriction. It is involved in pathophysiology of asthma.

3) Histamine stimulates nerve endings and produces itching.

4) Allergic or anaphylactic reactions are characterized by histamine release. The classical manifestations in allergies are due to above mentioned actions of histamine. Vasodilatation and exudation causes triple response: flush (red & then blue spot at the site of injection) flare (bright irregular outline up to 5 cm beyond flush) and wheal. It produces fall in blood pressure and bronchoconctriotion. Bronchoconstriction causes breathlessness. Stimulation of nerve endings by histamine causes itching.

5) Uterine and intestinal contractions induced by histamine are not very significant.

6) Adrenal medulla: Histamine promotes release of catecholamines from adrenal medulla and produces effects that are opposite to usual effects, i.e increase in BP.

Actions of histamine through H_2 receptors

The major action of histamine that is governed by only H_2 receptors is increased secretion of gastric HCL. Additionally, histamine also promotes secretion of pepsin. Thus histamine plays a crucial role in acidity and acid peptic disorders.

Histamine is a mediator in acid peptic disorders

Stimulation of H_2 receptors also produces vasodilatation (like H_1 receptors) and increase in rate and force of contraction of heart.

H_3 receptors: Their stimulation leads to inhibition of histamine secretion. They regulate histamine secretion.

Therapeutic uses

Histamine is not used clinically for therapeutic purposes. It is degraded immediately if given by oral route. In experimental studies histamine is used to induce acid release or for induction of bronchoconstriction.

Histamine is not used for any therapeutic purpose.

Drugs which act by modifying histaminergic action

1) Some drugs prevent release of histamine from mast cells and reduce histaminergic activity. Ex. Sodium cromoglycate.

2) Some drugs block histamine receptors and prevent effects of histamine. Ex. H_1 antagonists ('Conventional antihistaminics' or antiallergics), H_2 antagonists (acid reducing agents)

H_1 receptor antagonists or conventional antihistaminics

Antihistaminics is the term conventionally used for the agents, which block only H_1 receptors and not H_2. Agents from this class are widely used in clinical practice. Large number of antihistaminics are available for therapeutic purposes. Effectivitywise they are more or less same. It is the sedation (a common side effect) that differentiates these agents.

The term antihistaminic is conventionally used for the agents that block H_1 receptors.

Figure 3.3 Antihistaminic agents

Antihistaminic agents

Highly sedative	Moderately sedative	Less sedatives
Diphenhydramine	Cyproheptadine	Chlorpheniramine
Dimenhydrinate	Meclizine	Cyclizine
Promethazine	Pheniramine	Clemastine

Non sedative
- Astemizole
- Turfenadine
- Cetirizine
- Loratidine
- Azelastine
- Cinnarizine

Sedation is the major side effect of antihistaminic agents.

Nonsedative antihistaminics poorly penetrate blood brain barrier.

Mechanism of action

These agents competitively block H_1 receptors at various sites and prevent action of histamine. Therefore the effects are opposite to that of histamines. Antihistaminic agents produce bronchodilatation, prevent vasodilatation, reduce allergic skin reaction like flush, flair and wheal, prevent itching and prevent fall in BP. These actions are adequate enough to counter attack some allergic manifestations but not sufficient in anaphylactic reactions.

Some antihistaminic agents additionally can block cholinergic and serotonergic (5HT) receptors and produce additional actions. Anticholinergic action reduces salivary secretions and respiratory secretions. Reduction in mucus secretion helps in allergic respiratory disorder. Anticholinergic action also help in reducing cough and vomiting. Gastric acid secretion is controlled by H_2 receptors and is not inhibited by these agents.

Pharmacokinetics

These agents can be used orally as well as parenterally. They are metabolized in liver and excreted through kidney. Average duration of these agents is around 6 hours but some are longer acting. Sedation caused by these agents is decided by their penetration into brain. Non-sedative agents are poorly penetrated through blood brain barrier.

Indications

Allergic reactions: Antihistaminics (by preventing histamine mediated vasodilatation and increased permeability) reduce edema, rash and redness. They also block histamine induced stimulation of nerves and reduce itching and are used in pruritus, urticaria and nonspecific allergic reactions.

Anaphylaxis: Antihistaminics are commonly used as second line agents (with adrenaline or steroids) in anaphylactic reactions. Histamine mediated bronchoconstriction and vasodilatation is partly counteracted by these agents.

Common cold: These agents are effective in common cold due to their antihistaminic as well as anticholinergic activity. They reduce nasal congestion, nasal secretions, sneezing and nasal irritation that is associated with common cold. Sedation, a side effect, works as an advantage in children with common cold.

Cough: Antihistaminics have no action on the cough centre. But due to anticholinergic actions they reduce secretions, cause sedation and reduce cough.

Vomiting: Drug induced or post operative vomiting and motion sickness respond well to antihistaminics. The effect is governed by anticholinergic action of these drugs in CNS. Promethazine or cyclizine are commonly used as antiemetic agents.

Vertigo: Anticholinergic and anti5HT properties of these agents are helpful in vertigo. Cinnarizine is a preferred agent for vertigo.

Promethazine, cyclizine and meclizine are used in motion sickness.

Cinnarizine is used in vertigo.

Hay fever: It is a seasonal form of allergic rhinitis and is characterized by itching, swelling of nasal mucosa, sneezing, lacrimation, etc. Antiallergic actions of antihistaminics provide relief in hay fever.

Bronchial asthma: Histamine is not the only mediator involved in pathophysiology of asthma. Blocking of H_1 receptors does not give sufficient relief. Antihistaminics are used as second or third line agents in refractory asthma.

Preanesthetic medication: Promethazine, due to its anticholinergic action, reduces GI secretions and prevents chances of aspiration during anesthesia.

Antihistaminic agents are used to control dyskinetic movements in parkinsonism.

Adverse effects

Sedation is the most common side effect. Fatigue, drowsiness, light headedness, insomnia, nervousness, dry mouth and blurred vision are some other side effects.

Drug interactions

Sedation is potentiated when these agents are used along with alcohol or psychotropic drugs. These agents are usually avoided in breast feeding and pregnancy.

Individual antihistaminics are discussed in table 3.1

Table 3.1 Antihistaminic agents

Individual agents and dose	Features
Diphenhydramine 25-50 mg oral	Prototype agent Commonly used in respiratory disorders. Highly sedative but commonly used.
Chlorpheniramine CPM 2-4 mg oral, IM	Most commonly used antihistaminic Less sedation
Promethazine 25 mg oral IM Cyclizine 50 mg oral Meclizine 25-50 mg oral	Prominent anticholinergic activity. Mainly used as antiemetic agent or as preanesthetic medication to reduce secretions
Cinnarizine 25-50 mg oral	It has antihistaminic, anticholinergic and anti 5HT properties and by its action on labyrinth it is mainly used in vertigo.
Cyproheptadine 4 mg oral	It blocks histaminic, cholinergic and 5HT receptors. Along with antiallergic actions, it produces improvement in appetite and weight gain (most probably by its action (Cont.)

Cyproheptadine acts on various receptors and is used as an appetizer and anti-allergic agent.

	on growth hormone). Commonly used as appetite stimulant, antimigraine agent and antiallergic agent
Terfenadine 60-180 mg	Non-sedative and shorter acting. Severe cardiac toxicity due to interactions with macrolides (like erythromycin) and some antifungal agents (like ketoconazole).
Astemizole 10 mg oral	Non-sedative and long acting. No immediate relief. Cardiotoxic interactions similar to terfenadine.
Loratidine 10 mg oral	Non-sedative and long acting. Without cardiotoxic interactions like terfenadine.
Cetirizine 10 mg oral	Non sedative and long acting. Also prevents release of histamine from mast cells. Used in asthma also.
Azelastine 4 mg oral, nasal spray	Antihistaminic activity. Reduce histamine release. Additional antiinflammatory activity. Topically effective. Immediate relief.

The major problem with newer antihistaminics is their cardiotoxic interaction with some drugs.

Status

Antihistaminics are widely used agents for allergic disorders. Some agents have added anticholinergic and anti 5HT activity. Sedation is the major adverse effect; but newer agents produce less sedation.

5 Hydroxytryptamine (5HT) or serotonin

It is an amine autacoid, maximally present in mast cells of intestines, brain and platelets.

Synthesis and metabolism

Tryptophan is the precursor of 5HT. After formation it is usually not in free form in plasma but taken up by nerve endings and platelets.

5HT or Serotonin is predominantly present in brain and platelets.

Figure 3.4 Synthesis and metabolism of 5HT

Tryptophan
↓ ← Hydroxylase
5-Hydroxytryptophan
↓ ← decarboxylase
5HT
↓
Taken up in nerve endings and platelets and stored in storage granules
↓ ← Stimulus
Release of 5HT and Stimulation of 5HT (serotonergic) receptors
↓
Various actions
↓ ← MAO (monoaminooxidase/dehydrogenase)
Degradation products.

Mechanism of action of 5HT

Actions of 5HT are mediated through 5HT receptors. There are different families of 5HT receptor like $5HT_1$, $5HT_2$, $5HT_3$ up to $5HT_7$. There are subfamilies like $5HT_{1A}$, $5HT_{1B}$, $5HT_{1C}$, etc. Different receptors regulate different actions and there is a complex interplay in these actions. All receptors except $5HT_3$ are G protein coupled receptors and work through cyclic AMP or IP_3/DAG mechanism. $5HT_3$ receptors function by altering channel sensitivity.

Actions of 5HT

1) Brain: 5HT is a major neurotransmitter in brain that regulates sleep, temperature, mood variation, vomiting and pain. 5HT mediated vasoconstriction governs the initial stage of migraine. Cytotoxic drugs and radiotherapy induce vomiting through 5HT receptors in the brain.

2) 5HT, in platelets, promote aggregation of platelets and clotting.

3) Stimulation of 5HT receptors in GI tract alter motility of intestines and improve peristalsis. Additionally there is reduction in acid and pepsin.

4) CVS: Effects of 5HT on CVS are complex. They are mediated by different mechanisms that are given below:

i) Vascular dilatation through release of EDRF (Endothelium Dependant Relaxing Factor).

ii) Vasoconstriction through release of adrenaline from adrenal medulla.

iii) Vasoconstriction through action on autonomic ganglion.

iv) Sudden release of 5HT causes vasospastic episodes.

Due to above metioned actions a typical triphasic response is observed after IV administration of 5HT.

a) Initial reduction in BP

b) Immediate rise in BP

c) Sustained reduction in BP

5HT is believed to be involved in allergy, inflammation, carcinoid tumor, etc.

Therapeutic application

5HT is not used clinically.

5HT is not used clinically. Modification of serotonergic system by various drugs offer significant clinical advantages.

Drugs that alter storage or transport of 5HT

Fluoxetine, Trazodone: antidepressants

Fenfluramine: anorectic

5HT agonists: Following drugs, like 5HT stimulate 5HT receptors and produce similar actions.

Buspirone: antianxiety

Sumatriptan: antimigraine (Refer page 134).

Cisapride: prokinetic agent (Refer page 209).

Methysergide: It is a partial agonist and antagonist of 5HT receptors. It has peripheral antagonistic and central agonistic action on 5HT receptor. Additionally it has a vasoconstrictor action. It is used for prophylaxis of migraine but has got no role once attack is established. (Dose: 1- 2 mg BD-TID).

Side effects - GI disturbances, hypotension, tachycardia, etc.

5HT antagonists

These drugs block 5HT receptors and prevent actions of 5HT. Many agents like α blockers or antihistaminics have anti5HT activity, but following agents have selective activity in different disorders.

Table 3.2 5HT antagonist

i) In schizophrenia	Clozapine Risperidone
ii) In vomiting	Ondansetron Granisetron
iii) In migraine prophylaxis	Methysergide Pizotifen
iv) In hypertension and Raynaud's disease	Ketanserin

Cyproheptadine has got anti5HT properties. (Refer page 122).

Methysergide has both agonistic and antagonistic actions on 5HT receptors and is used for prophylaxis of migraine.

Plasma kinins

These are peptide autacoids and these include bradykinin and kallidin. They are generally produced in response to injuries or due to contact of some negatively charged substances.

Synthesis and release

Kinins are derived from kininogens. Kininogens are of two types-high molecular weight (HMW) and low molecular weight (LMW). The formation of kinins from these kininogens is stimulated by injury. Injury results in activation of clotting factor XII (Hageman factor). This activated factor XII converts prokallikrein into kallikrein. These kallikreins are either tissue kallikrein or plasma kallikreins. These are responsible for production of kinins.

Figure 3.5 Synthesis and release of kinins

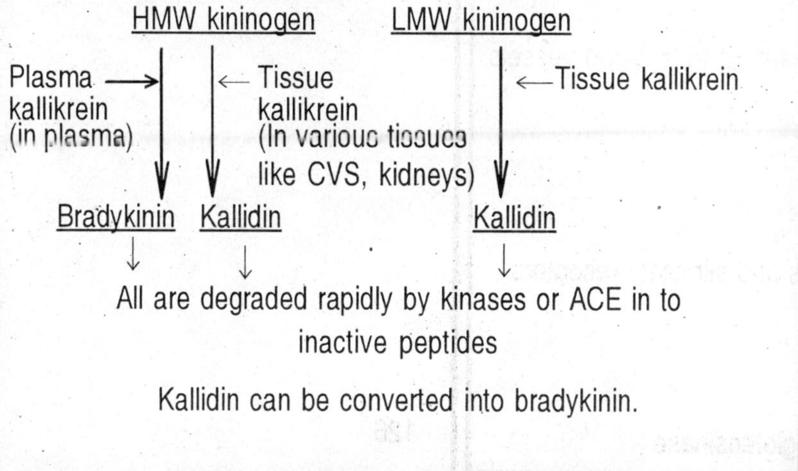

Actions and roles of kinins

Both kinins, bradykinin and kallidin, have similar action which is mediated through B_1 and B_2 receptors. These are G protein coupled receptors and their action is mediated through IP_3/DAG. Additionally, kinins induce release of histamine, PAF, PGs, etc. Kinins have following physiological roles:

1) **Inflammatory response:** Kinins through release of EDRF (endothelium dependant relaxing factors) produce vasodilatation and cause increase in blood flow at the site of injury. Increased permeability produces exudation and stimulation of pain receptor produces pain. Thus inflammatory process is mediated through kinins.

Kinins are mediators in process of inflammation, pain and allergy.

2) Independent of inflammation, kinins act as mediators of pain by stimulating nerve endings.

3) Kinins are also mediators in allergy and asthma.

4) Dilatation of vessels can produce fall in BP.

5) Kinins contract smooth muscles of GI tract and that of bronchi.

6) Kinins also play some role in

i) Clotting and fibrinolytic system

ii) Establishment of neonatal circulation

iii) Microcirculation of kidneys

Kinins are not used therapeutically

Angiotensin

Angiotensin is a peptide autacoid that is involved especially in cardiovascular regulation of body. Modification in angiotensin activity is used widely in clinical practices.

Synthesis and metabolism: Angiotensin production is governed by Renin Angiotensin system. The system is present in many organs in the body: viz. kidney, heart, blood vessels, brain, etc.

Figure 3.6 Synthesis and metabolism

Angiotensinogen (Inactive precursor)
↓ ← Renin from plasma
Angiotensin I (Inactive)
↓ ← Angiotensin Converting Enzyme (ACE) from blood vessels
Angiotensin II (active)
↓ ← Aminopeptidases
Angiotensin III
↓
A II and A III get attached to AT receptors and stimulate receptors
↓
Various actions
↓
Angiotensin is degraded by enzyme angiotensinase

Regulation of angiotensin is governed by secretion of renin. The regulation of Renin Angiotensin system is done in following manner.

Renin-angiotensin system is predominantly involved in regulation of blood pressure.

- ✦ Reduction in blood pressure,
- ✦ Reduction in renal blood flow,
- ✦ Reduction in plasma Na concentration

↓

Increased activity of renin

↓

Activation of Renin Angiotensin system

↓

Formation of angiotensin

↓

Increase in renal blood flow, rise in BP and increase in Na concentration.

↓

Reduced renin secretion

↓

These effects are produced as follows:

Actions and roles of angiotensin

Effects of angiotensin are mediated through AT_1 and AT_2 receptors. These are G protein coupled receptors. Their actions are governed through IP_3/DAG.

Action on blood vessels

Angiotensin II increases BP by increasing PR and retaining urinary Na and water.

Angiotensin has two major actions on blood vessels.

i) Increased central sympathetic outflow

ii) Increased release of adrenaline and NA from adrenal medulla and nerve endings.

Both these actions produce increase in peripheral resistance and blood pressure. As a long term effects it produces growth of arterial walls.

Action on heart

Angiotensin II causes hypertrophy of arterial walls and heart.

Direct action of angiotensin on heart produces increase in the force of contraction of heart but reflex parasympathetic activation (due to rise in peripheral resistance) reduces that. Additionally, angiotensin has got direct action on heart that causes hypertrophy.

Action on adrenal cortex

Angiotensin stimulates release of aldosterone from adrenal cortex. Aldosterone retains water and Na and increases fluid volume in body

Action on kidneys

Angiotensin II increases Na and Cl reabsorption directly. The effect is independent of aldosterone.

Angiotensin II is involved in pathophysiology of cardiac and diabetic renal disorders.

Angiotensins are not therapeutically used. Different modifications in Renin Angiotensin system provide therapeutic benefits.

Ex. i) Renin specific antibodies reduce renin activity
ii) ACE inhibitors reduce formation of A II (Refer page 138).
iii) Angiotensin II blockers block AT receptors (Refer page 141).

Lipid derived autacoids

Figure 3.7 Lipid derived autacoids

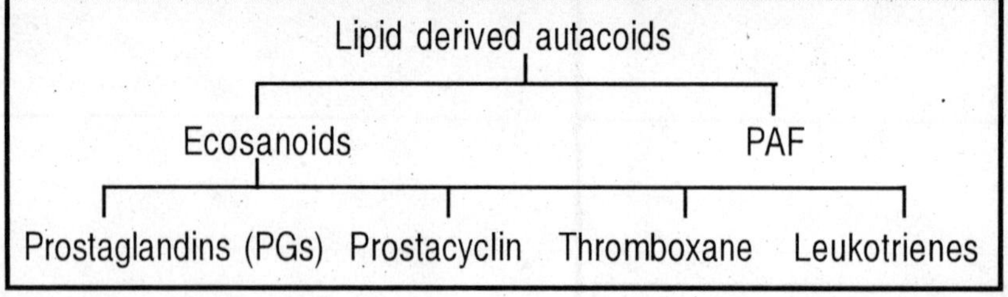

Ecosanoids

Ecosanoids are the autacoids that are derived from arachidonic acid and include prostaglandins (PGs), prostacyclin (PGI), Thromboxanes (TX) and leukotreines (LT). They are widely distributed in the body and almost all cells in the body produce some of these ecosanoids. PGs are classified as PGE, PGF, PGG, PGH, etc. Similarly leukotrienes are classified as LTA_4, LTB_4, LTC_4, etc. Thromboxanes are of types TXA_2 and TXB_2. Release of phospholipase A_2 from the site of injury stimulates the cascade of production of all ecosanoids.

Figure 3.8 Synthesis and release of ecosanoids

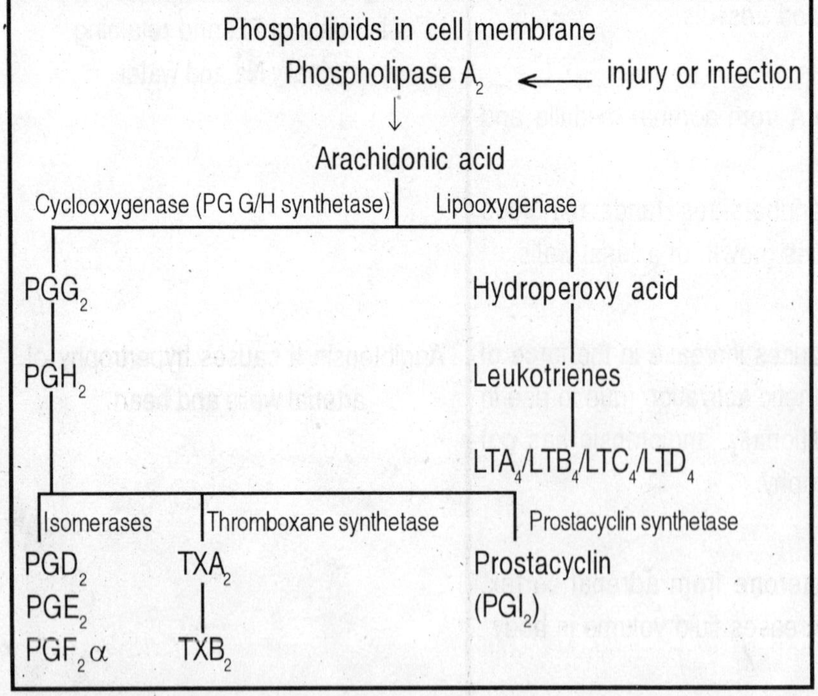

Prostaglandins and prostacycline

The name prostaglandin (PG) is derived from the fact that they are initially extracted from prostate. PGs are predominantly present in seminal fluid, lungs, brain, pancreas etc. But almost all cells can produce PGs.

Synthesis and release: Refer figure 3.8

Mechanism of action

These agents act on respective receptors like PGD on DP, PGE on EP, PGF on FP and prostacyclines of IP.

All these receptors are G protein coupled and their actions are mediated through IP_3/DAG mediated mechanism.

Actions and roles of PGs

Inflammation: PGs are major inflammatory mediators. They have following actions at the site of inflammation.

i) Dilatation of blood vessels - Redness

ii) Increased capillary permeability - Exudation

iii) Sensitisation of pain receptors - Pain.

PGs are involved in pathophysiology of inflammation, diarrhea, platelet aggregation, dysmenorrhea, acid peptic disorders, fever, etc.

Gastroprotection: PGs have following protective actions on GI tract,

i) Reduced acid secretion

ii) Increased mucus formation

iii) Improvement in gastric blood flow

PGs, additionally govern intestinal motility and secretions and probably are involved in regulation of diarrhoea.

Bronchial muscles: Some PGs cause bronchodilatation while some cause bronchoconstriction. But bronchodilator effect is predominant.

CNS: PGs, through their action on hypothalamus, regulate body temperature and are involved in pathophysiology of fever.

Kidneys

PGs produce diuretic effect by reducing Na^+, K^+ and water reabsorption. They also maintains renal blood flow.

Uterus

PGs contract uterus and the sensitivity of uterus for PGs is increased in pregnancy. Hence, PGs are thought to be the mediators of dysmenorrhea (painful menstruations). PGs are also involved in progression of labor.

CVS

PGs produce mainly vasodilatation and cause fall in BP but some PGs produce vasoconstriction. They have weak positive inotropic action. PGs maintain patency of ductus arteriosus in fetal life and during birth. Reduction in PGs facilitates closure of ductus arteriosus.

Platelets

PGs and thromboxanes together govern platelet aggregation and anti aggregation. Some PGs and TXs produce platelet aggregation while PGI inhibits aggregation.

Clinical applications

Therapeutic advantages are achieved either by administration of PG derivatives or by inhibiting actions of prostaglandins.

Therapeutic uses of PGs

Prostaglandin derivatives are used in variety of clinical conditions.

Misoprostol (PGE_1): It is used in peptic ulcer and it protects GI mucosa by reducing acid secretion, increasing mucus secretion and improving circulation.

Dinoprostone (PGE): This agent is used to induce labor. It stimulates uterine contractions. It is also used in inducing abortions. It is available in intravenous form or vaginal gel.

Carboprost ($PGF_2\alpha$): It is used to reduce post-partum hemorrhage. It acts by inducing uterine contractions.

Alprostadil (PGE1): It maintains patency of ductus arteriosus in neonates having cardiac disorders (till surgery is undertaken).

PGI_2 Epoprostenol: It prevents platelet aggregation during hemodialysis.

Drugs acting by inhibiting PGs

Nonsteroidal antiinflammatory drugs (NSAIDs) inhibit enzyme cyclooxygenase, and inhibit formation of PGs and TX and inhibit the process of inflammation. But inhibition of PGs at GI, kidney and respiratory tract causes adverse effects like GI disturbance, NSAID induced asthma and nephrotoxicity. Now it is proved that enzyme cyclooxygenase (COX) exists in two different types COX I and COX II.

NSAIDs like aspirin, ibuprofen, diclofenac produce effects by inhibiting PG synthesis

COX I - It produces PGs that are involved in noninflammatory activities like GI, respiratory and renal protection.

COX II - It produces PGs that are involved in process of inflammation.

Newer NSAIDs inhibit enzyme COX-II selectively and reduce side effects

Newer NSAIDs like nimesulide, rofecoxib and celecoxib inhibit only one type of cyclooxygenase (COX II) and inhibit formation of pro-inflammatory prostaglandins but do not affect protective prostaglandins. These agents are safer compared to previous agents.

Thromboxanes (TX)

Thromboxanes are lipid derived autacoids and are ecosanoids. They are not as extensively distributed as PGs. They are of two types: TXA_2 and TXB_2.

Synthesis and release :

TXs are synthesized from arachidonic acid and the synthesis has already been discussed (Refer Figure 3.8, Page 128).

Mechanism of action

TXs act on TP receptors. These are G proteins coupled receptors and their action is mediated by IP_3/DAG mechanism.

Actions and roles of TXs

TXs are mainly involved in platelet aggregation and release reaction during injuries. TXs are also mediators in bronchial asthma as they produce bronchoconstriction. TXs produce contraction of intestinal smooth muscles.

Thromboxanes are involved in pathophysiology of platelet aggregation and bronchial asthma.

Therapeutic application

TXs are not used therapeutically, but modification in their action produces therapeutic advantages. Aspirin, in low doses, prevents TX formation and prevents platelet aggregation in MI or cerebrovascular disorders.

Antiplatelet action of aspirin is mediated through inhibition of thromboxane synthesis

Leukotrienes (LTs)

These are lipid derived autacoids and are ecosanoids. LTA_4, LTB_4, LTC_4, LTD_4 are different subtypes of LTs.

Synthesis and release:

LTs are synthesized from arachidonic acid and the synthesis has already been discussed (Refer Figure 3.8, Page 128).

Mechanism of action

LTs stimulate specific LT receptors. They are G protein coupled receptors and their actions are mediated through IP_3/DAG.

Actions and roles

LTs are involved in pathophysiology of inflammation, asthma and rheumatoid arthritis.

1) LTs act on coronary vessels and cause coronary constriction. It leads to decreased cardiac blood flow and subsequent reduction in CO and BP.

2) Inflammation: LTs increase capillary permeability and cause exudation of fluids. LTs act as chemotactic factors and attract neutrophils and promote process of inflammation. LTs also sensitize nerve endings and produce pain sensation. LTs stimulate proliferation of T lymphocytes and cause release of lysozymes from neutrophils.

3) LTs cause bronchoconstriction and increase mucus secretion in respiratory tract. Thus they are involved in pathophysiology of asthma.

Platelet Activating Factor (PAF)

PAF is lipid derived autacoid but not ecosanoid. It is produced by limited number of cells mainly WBCs, platelets, vascular cells and kidney.

Synthesis and release

Figure 3.9 Synthesis and release of PAF

Phospholipids in cell membranes

↓← Phospholipase A_2 ← Injury

Lyso PAF

↓← PAF acetyltransferase

PAF

↓

Gets attached to PAF receptors and stimulates receptors (IP_3/DAG mediated mechanism)

↓

Various actions

↓

Degradation

Actions and roles

1) Inflammation and allergies:

PAF produces dilatation of blood vessels and causes exudation, swelling, redness, wheel and flair. It also acts as chemotactic factor and attracts neutrophils and promote process of inflammation and allergy.

PAF is involved in pathophysiology of inflammation, allergy, bronchial asthma and anaphylactic shock.

2) Anaphylactic reaction is also partly mediated by PAF. PAF produces EDRF mediated vasodilatation.

3) PAF is a mediator in bronchial asthma due to its bronchoconstricting action.

4) It stimulates platelet aggregation and release reaction.

5) PAF has got ulcerogenic action.

Therapeutic application

PAF is not used therapeutically but drugs that block PAF receptors (PAF antagonists) are used for prevention of platelet aggregation, asthma and peptic ulcer

Cytokines

Cytokines are autacoids involved in the immunological and inflammatory processes. They play a major role in human defence. Cytokines are produced by variety of cells, predominantly WBCs. They are also involved in growth and differentiation of WBCs. Some of the cytokines have action on viral cells. Cytokines include - Interferons, Colony Stimulating Factors (CSF), Interleukins, Tumor Necrosis Factor (TNFα).

Interferons

These are glycoprotein cytokines. The cells in body that are infected by viruses naturally produce interferons. But they do not have specificity for viruses. Each species produces different types of interferons.

Interferons are produced by virus infected cells in the body.

i) Alpha interferon
ii) Beta interferon
iii) Gamma interferon

All these interferons are manufactured by gene recombination technology and are used therapeutically.

Mechanism of action

Interferons induce direct degradation of viral DNA and affect viral replication in different ways. Additionally, interferons alter host immunity by improving activity of T lymphocytes and macrophages.

Interferons are used therapeutically in viral infections, leukemia and multiple sclerosis.

Therapeutic applications of interferons

i) Cancers: α interferon is effective in various cancers like leukemia, renal carcinoma, kaposis sarcoma in AIDS and also in genital worts.

ii) Alpha interferon is also effective in hepatitis B and C (5 million units/

day SC or IM over a period of 6 months is effective in hepatitis B).

iii) β interferon, when used in multiple sclerosis, reduces intervals between relapses and improve physical performance of patient.

Side effects

Flu like syndrome: Fever, chills, headache fatigue, anorexia. Long term toxicity includes weight loss, bone marrow depression, anemia and arrhythmias.

Colony Stimulating Factors (CSFs)

Colony Stimulating Factors promote production and differentiation of WBCs.

CSFs are cytokine type of autacoids. They are involved in growth and multiplication of WBCs. CSFs are used therapeutically to induce growth of WBCs.

Mechanism of action

These agents stimulate growth, differentiation and activity of colonies of myeloid cells.

Therapeutic application

Filgrastim and lenograstim: They are granulocyte colony stimulating factors (GCSF). These drugs stimulate maturation and proliferation of neutrophils and are administered by intravenous infusion or subcutaneous route.

Molgramostim: This is GMCSF i.e. granulocyte macrophage colony stimulating factor. It has effect on granulocytes as well as monocytes and it is administered by IV infusion or SC route.

Both these drugs are indicated in idiopathic neutropenia, neutropenia due to cancer therapy, after bone marrow transplantation, aplastic anemia and AIDS.

Adverse effects : Common side effect include bone and muscle pain, splenomegaly and allergic reactions.

Interleukins

Interleukins and TNF are involved in inflammation, repair and killing of organisms and host defence.

These are cytokine types of autacoids. They are mainly produced by T cells, monocytes and macrophages. They are of various types ranging from IL1 to IL7.

Actions

1) Interleukins stimulate proliferation of T lymphocytes and activate natural killer cells.
2) ILs promote migration of defence cell at the site of inflammation.
3) ILs kill various organisms
4) ILs play major role in repair of the wounds.

Therapeutic applications

Interleukin 2, when given therapeutically, is effective in renal carcinoma and malignant melanoma and blocking of IL2 in rheumatoid arthritis provides relief.

Cytotoxic factors: Tumor Necrosis Factor α (TNFα)

This is a cytokine autacoid and is cytotoxic. It is responsible for destruction of tumor cells. TNF induces production of free radicals and kills organisms. TNF, like ILs, is responsible for repairing wounds. TNF is the mediator that causes destruction of bone matrix in rheumatoid arthritis. Antibody against it or blockade of TNF α receptors produce improvement in rheumatoid arthritis.

Management of migraine

Migraine is a throbbing pulsatile headache mostly on one side. It is most probably due to altered calibre of cranial blood vessels. It can be associated with nausea, vomiting, photophobia and diarrhoea. Aura is a subjective sensation that precedes before migraine. Classical migraine is a migraine with aura and nonclassical migraine is without aura. Various mediators involved in pathophysiology of migraine are 5HT, adrenaline, prostaglandins, substance P, etc.

Migraine can be associated with nausea, vomiting, photophobia and diarrhoea

Objectives of management

1) Reducing pain if attack is already established.
2) Preventing attacks of migraine.

Nonpharmacological management

Various factors like cheese, chocolates, smoking, stress, hunger, fatigue, sleep disturbances etc. provoke migraine. They must be avoided.

Pharmacological management

Figure 3.10 Drugs used in management of migraine

Drugs used in management of migraine

- For acute attack
  - NSAIDs: Aspirin, Ibuprofen, Ketorolac, Diclofenac
  - Ergots: Ergotamine, Dihydroergotamine
  - Caffeine
  - 5HT receptor agonists: Sumatriptan
  - Opioid analgesics: Codeine, Meperidine
  - Antiemetic: Metoclopramide
- For prophylaxis
  - β blockers: Propranolol
  - Calcium channel blockers: Flunarizine, Verapamil
  - 5HT antagonists: Methysergide, Pizotifen
  - Tricyclic antidepressants: Imipramine

Mechanism by which drugs act in migraine

NSAIDs: These drugs inhibit enzyme cyclooxygenase and reduce formation of prostaglandins and reduce pain. Paracetamol 500 mg or ibuprofen 400 mg are commonly used NSAIDs. In severe cases ketorolac IM 15-30 mg every 4-6 hrs (max 120 mg/day) is used.

Opioid analgesics: These drugs act on opioid receptors in CNS and reduce pain. They are commonly used in moderate or severe migraine, that is not controlled by NSAIDs.
Codeine 30-60 mg oral, Meperidine 50-150 mg oral

Opioids are used in resistant cases

Ergot derivatives: These agents have complex actions on blood vessels. They are:
Partial agonists of α receptors
Partial agonists of 5HT receptors
Antagonists of β_2 receptors.

Their vascular actions are mainly responsible for relief in migraine. Ergotamine and dihydroergotamine are commonly used ergots in migraine. Ergotamine is more potent. It is best effective if administered in prodromal stage (aura). These agents have no prophylactic value.

Ergotamine is best effective if administered in prodromal stage.

Ergotamine: Start with 2-3 mg oral dose. 1-2 mg can be given every 30 minutes till relief: max 10 mg. In case of vomiting SC or rectal route is preferred.

Dihydroergotamine: It is used in refractory cases. 1-2 mg SC or IV.

Caffeine: Caffeine is a xanthine alkaloid and potentiates effects of ergotamine or NSAIDs. It acts as an analgesic adjuvant.

Sumatriptan: It produces action by stimulating 5HT receptors on blood vessels. It has side effects like nausea, vomiting, tightness in chest, arrhythmias and is contraindicated in heart diseases. In migraine, if ergotamine is a co-treatment, it should be administered 6 hours after sumatriptan and next sumatriptan should be administered 24 hours after ergotamine. Dose: 50-100 mg oral, 6 mg SC.

Antiemetics: As migraine usually is associated with vomiting, metoclopramide (10 mg oral or IM) or prochlorperazine (10-20 mg oral or IM) is used to prevent vomiting.

Prophylactic agents

β blockers: Propranolol (20 mg BD-oral up to 160 mg BD) can prevent attacks of migraine. The action is mediated through blockade of β_2 receptors but still the exact machanism is not very clear.

Calcium channel blockers: These agents prevent entry of calcium into vascular cells and dilate blood vessels. But their effectivity is limited and are rarely used in migraine prophylaxis.

Tricyclic antidepressants: Mechanism of action of these agents in migraine is not clear, Amitriptyline (10-50 mg/day before sleeping) is most commonly used antidepressant for migraine.

5HT antagonists: Though 5HT agonists are used in migraine, paradoxically antagonists of 5HT receptors also provide protection in migraine. Methysergide (2 mg OD up to 8 mg).
Prednisolone (60-80 mg/day) are also effective in migraine prophylaxis.

Line of management for migraine

Figure 3.11 Acute attack of migraine

Acute attack

Mild
↓
Paracetamol
↓
If not controlled
↓
Ibuprofen
add metoclopramide if vomiting

Moderate
↓
Combination of NSAIDs/Opioids
or
Sumatriptan
or
Ergotamine + Caffeine
add metoclopramide if vomiting

Severe
↓
Parenteral ketorolac
or
Ergotamine + Caffeine
or
Sumatriptan
↓
add metoclopramide if vomiting

Prophylaxis

Nonpharmacological management (i.e. avoiding provocative factors) if is not sufficient and if there are 2 or more attacks in a month, any of the suitable agents are used for prophylaxis. Up to 3 months are required to get optimum effect. The drugs are gradually withdrawn after the su ccessful prevention of the disease. Amitriptyline or methysergide are drugs of choice for prophylaxis of migraine.

DRUGS IN CARDIOVASCULAR SYSTEM

"THIS SECTION CONTAINS"

ANGIOTENSIN CONVERTING ENZYME INHIBITORS
(ACE INHIBITORS)

It is a class of drugs that are widely used in variety of cardiovascular disorders as the first line therapy. Agents from this class are captopril, enalapril, lisinopril, benazepril, perindopril etc.

Physiological considerations: (Refer page 126).
Kidneys, heart, blood vessels, etc. contain a system called as renin angiotensin system. It is involved in regulating blood pressure. It works in following fashion

ACE inhibitors inhibit synthesis of angiotensin II

Figure 4.1 Effects of angiotensin

Angiotensinogen
↓ Renin ← Renin is released in response to fall in BP, reduction in blood volume and Na depletion.
Angiotensin I (Inert)
↓ ACE
Angiotensin II (AII) (active)
↓
Stimulates AT_1 receptors

<u>CVS</u>
Vasoconstriction
↓
↑ Peripheral resistance
↓
↑ Blood pressure
↓
<u>Long term effects</u>
Hypertrophy of arterial walls and that of heart muscles

<u>Adrenal cortex</u>
Synthesis and release of aldosterone
↑ Na and water retention

<u>Visceral smooth muscles</u>
Contraction

<u>Sympathomimetic action</u>
↑ in central sympathetic outflow
↑release of NA/Adr from adrenal medulla and nerve endings

ACE inhibitors: Mechanism of action

These drugs inhibit Angiotensin Converting Enzyme and prevent synthesis of A II. This offers following advantages:

i) Prevention of A II mediated vasoconstriction reduces peripheral resistance and blood pressure.

ii) Prevention of A II mediated synthesis of aldosterone reduces Na and water retention. There is reduction in fluid overload.

iii) Reduction in central symptomatic activity reduces sympathetic overactivity.

iv) Prevention of hypertrophy of heart and arterial walls.

ACE inhibitors
1.Reduce BP
2. Decrease fluid overload
3. Reduce sympathetic overactivity

v) Bradykinin is a vasodilator that is metabolized by ACE. ACE inhibitors prevent metabolism and degradation of bradykinin and bradykinin dilates blood vessels.

vi) ACE inhibitors produce improvement in kidney function and reduce microalbuminuria.

Actions of ACE inhibitors depend on activity of renin and plasma Na concentration. They produce maximum fall in BP when Na is depleted in renovascular hypertension. With ACE inhibitors, inactivation of sympathetic system is not a major mechanism that lowers BP. Therefore reduction in BP does not result in reflex sympathetic overactivity

Indications

Hypertension: ACE inhibitors are used as the first line agent in various subclasses of hypertensive patients. These drugs reduce BP by mainly vasodilatation (by inhibiting angiotensin mediated vasoconstriction and by protecting bradykinin).

ACE inhibitors reduce BP without reflex sympathetic stimulation.

Additionally by inhibiting aldosterone, these drugs reduce fluid overload. ACE inhibitors act on both arteries and veins and reduce both systolic and diastolic blood pressure. They do not produce postural hypotension. Renal, cerebral and coronary blood flow is not compromised by ACE inhibitors. ACE inhibitor reverse diabetic nephropathy and cardiac hypertrophy. These are the drugs of choice in hypertension associated with these two disorders.

ACE inhibitors are drugs of choice in renovascular hypertension and in hypertension associated with diabetic nephropathy and cardiac hypertrophy.

Heart failure: ACE inhibitors offer following advantages in heart failure:
i) Arterial dilatation reduces afterload
ii) Venous dilatation reduces preload
iii) Reduced retention of Na and water reduces fluid overload. Thus without direct action on heart, they (i) Reduce work load of heart, (ii) Produce improvement in stroke volume and (iii) Improve cardiac output (iv) Without increase in heart rate.

Myocardial infarction: ACE inhibitors, if administered within 24 hours and continued for 6 weeks, provide long-term protection in MI.

ACE inhibitors offer protection in diabetic nephropathy and end stage renal disorders in diabetes.

ACE inhibitors are teratogenic in the second half of pregnancy

Individual ACE inhibitors: (Refer table 4.1 page 140).
Precautions and interactions
1) These agents are not used in bilateral renal artery stenosis and in patients with known hypersensitivity to these drugs.
2) Diuretics are preferably stopped before giving ACE inhibitors because both the classes of drugs reduce fluid contents in the body.
3) NSAIDs blunt hypotensive action of ACE inhibitors

Adverse effects:

1) Inhibition of metabolism of bradykinin and substance P results in cough, a common side effects of ACE inhibitor. Cough may demand withdrawal of the drug.

2) There can be a sudden drop in blood pressure after first dose: first dose effect. Patients must be warned about it or first dose is given before sleeping.

3) Headache, dizziness, rash, loss of taste are some other side effects

4) ACE inhibitors are not given in acute renal failure as by dilating renal vessels, they can drop glomerular filtration pressure. This results in worsening of renal failure.

5) ACE inhibitors are teratogenic in second half of pregnancy.

Cough is a side effect of ACE inhibitors

First dose hypotension is common with ACE inhibitors

ACE inhibitors are contraindicated in pregnancy.

Table 4.1 ACE inhibitors

Agent and dose	Features
Captopril 25 mg BD-TDS up to 150 mg	Shortest acting. The only drug that is to be given in two to three doses.
Enalapril 5 mg OD (or 2.5) up to 40 mg	Prodrug-converted into active enalaprilat. More potent. Long acting. Less side effects like rash, change in taste Absorption not affected by food.
Lisinopril 5-10 mg OD up to 40 mg	Less chances of first dose effect. Long acting.
Ramipril 1.25, 2.5 mg OD up to 20 mg	Prodrug. Extensive distribution. Long acting.
Perindopril 2 mg OD up to 8 mg	Prodrug.
Benazepril 10-20 mg OD/BD up to 40 mg	

Status of ACE inhibitors

ACE inhibitors are the only vasodilators without reflex sympathetic activity. So they are effectively used in HT and heart failure. They are the drugs of choice in renovascular hypertension.

They are beneficially used in HT associated with diabetic nephropathy and left ventricular hypertrophy.

They can be combined with other antihypertensives. Cough can be a limiting factor to their use.

They do not have effects on lipid profile. They are contraindicated in second trimester of pregnancy and acute renal failure.

Angiotensin antagonist: Losartan

It selectively blocks angiotensin receptors and produces actions very similar to ACE inhibitors. But it does not have same side effects.

Losartan doesn't inhibit enzyme ACE but it blocks AT receptors.

Mechanism of action

It selectively blocks AT_1 receptors and prevents stimulation of these receptors by angiotensin. It does not have any action on formation of A II, like ACE inhibitors. It produces:

1) Vasodilatation and reduces PR and BP
2) Inhibition of central sympathetic tone
3) Blocks release of adrenaline
4) Inhibits Na and water retention in kidney and reduces fluid overload and preload.

All these actions are responsible for reduction in peripheral resistance and reduced oxygen demand of heart. Losartan is used in hypertension. Its uses in CCF and other cardiovascular conditions are under investigation.
Dose: 25-50 mg oral OD or BD

Adverse effects

The major advantage with losartan is that, like ACE inhibitors, it has no effect on bradykinin and so it does not produce cough. But hypokalemia, headache, GI disturbances are the side effects that are similar to ACE inhibitors. It is contraindicated in pregnancy.

Unlike ACE inhibitors, losartan doesn't produce cough.

Calcium channel blockers (CCBs)

Physiological considerations

Calcium influx in cells is essential for contraction of cardiac and vascular cells. Entry of calcium in cells is governed by three types of channels.

i) Voltage sensitive channels.
ii) Receptor operated channels.
iii) Leak channels.

Voltage sensitive channels get activated when there is a drop in membrane potential. Voltage sensitive channels are of three types L, N and T.

Calcium Channel Blockers

CCBs are widely used drugs in cardiovascular disorders. They are classified as:

Dihydropyridines: Nifedipine, amlodipine, nimodipine, nicardipine, felodipine. Nifedipine is first generation drug and all the others are from second generation.
Benzothiazepine: Diltiazem
Phenylalkylamines: Verapamil

Mechanism of action

CCBs produce their effects by blocking entry of calcium in cells. CCBs inhibit L type of voltage sensitive Ca channels.

(Refer figure 4.2)

CCBs block L type of voltage sensitive calcium channels

Figure 4.2 Mechanism of action of CCBs

CCBs
↓
Prevent entry of Ca through L channels
↓
↓ influx of Ca
↓
↓ intracellular Ca
↓
No contraction of various smooth muscles

Arterial dilatation ↓ ↓ PR ↓ ↓ BP Dilatation of pulmonary arteries	↓ Force of contraction of heart ↓ Rate of heart ↓ Conduction Dilatation of coronary blood vessels	Smooth muscle relaxation ↓ Bronchodilatation Biliary tract dilatation Dilatation of GI smooth muscles.

CCBs act on arteries, heart and some other smooth muscles.

Pharmacokinetics

These drugs are administered by oral, sublingual or injectable routes. They are well absorbed from GIT. Agents from dihydropyridine class undergo first pass effect

Indications

Angina pectoris

CCBs are not used as the first line management therapy for angina but they usually are administered along with nitrates or β blockers. CCBs, by dilating arteries, reduce afterload and decrease oxygen demand of heart. By dilating coronary blood vessels, CCBs offer relief in variant angina. These agents are also used in unstable angina (Refer page 170).

Hypertension

CCBs reduce blood pressure mainly by dilating arteries and reducing peripheral resistance. CCBs are used as the first line drugs in management of systemic and pulmonary hypertension and can be combined with different antihypertensive. (Refer page 177). CCBs are drugs of choice in HT with COPD, asthma and peripheral vascular disorders.

CCBs are drugs of choice in HT with COPD, asthma and peripheral vascular disorders.

Cardiac dysrrhythmias: Verapamil is the only (rarely diltiazem) agent that has sufficient action on heart to improve arrhythmia, especially supraventricular arrhythmias, atrial flutter and fibrillation.

Cardiac failure: Role of CCBs in cardiac failure is controversial and limited.

Peripheral vascular disorders: These disorders are characterized by peripheral vascular spasm. CCBs, by dilating blood vessels, provide relief in peripheral spasm.

CCBs are occasionally used in prophylaxis of migraine. Ischemic neurological damage after subarachinoid hemorrhage can be prevented by CCBs. These drugs also act as uterine relaxants.

Individual agents

All agents have action on blood vessels. So agents mainly are differentiated by their action on heart. Dihydropyridines are more potent with less action on heart.

Dihydropyridines (Nifedipine like drugs) predominantly act on arteries while verapamil has more action on heart. Diltiazem lies in-between.

Table 4.2 Calcium channel blockers

Agent and dose	Features
Nifedipine 10-30 mg TDS/QID Slow release 30-120 mg OD Sublingual 10 mg	First generation CCB Less effect on heart Undergoes first pass effect Effective in hypertensive emergency Reflex increase in heart rate is possible
Amlodipine 2.5 to 10 mg OD	Long acting: continued protection Less first pass effect Slow acting: so early adverse effects of vasodilatation are avoided. Safe in cardiac patient and now a choice in hypertension.
Nicardipine 20-40 mg TDS 30-60 mg SR BD	--
Diltiazem 30-90 mg OD 180-360 mg OD extended release	Effect on heart is (-ve inotropic, -ve dromotropic and -ve chronotrpic) more than dihydropyridines but less than verapamil. Effect is compensated by reflex sympathetic stimulation and tachycardia.
Verapamil IV 10 mg over 2-3 minutes. 40-80 mg oral TDS-QID	Major action on heart. Used in arrhythmia. Can precipitate CCF. Should not be given if patient is having bradycardia. Not administered with β blockers. It has got some α blocking action.

Amlodipine, a long acting dihydropyridine, is a preferred agent in hypertension.

Beta-blockers are not used with verapamil but can be used with nifedipine.

Verapamil is used in arrhythmias.

Felodipine, lacidipine, isradipine are some additional CCBs from dihydropyridine class.

Adverse effects

Headache, flushing, dizziness, edema, postural hypotension, etc. are the side effects produced due to vasodilatation. Palpitations may be due to reflex sympathetic stimulation. Nausea, vomiting, constipation are some additional side effects.

Precautions and interactions

1) Use of verapamil and diltiazem should be avoided along with β-blockers. (as both these classes inhibit cardiac function)

2) These drugs are used with caution in hepatic and renal impairment.

Status

These are the first line drugs in hypertension. They are used in angina along with β blockers and nitrates, CCBs are useful in situations where β blockers are contraindicated. Nifedipine is a preferred agent in pregnancy, renal hypertension and diabetes.

NITRATES

Physiological considerations

Nitric oxide (NO) is a natural vasodilator in human body. It is produced by endothelial cells and is responsible mainly for dilatation of veins. To some extent it also dilates arteries.

Nitrates

Basically nitrates are used in explosives. Tablets, if are exposed to heat or air, lose their potency due to evaporation. They are drugs of choice in angina pectoris.

Mechanism of action:

Nitrates act in body by releasing NO (Refer figure 4.3 on page 145).

Pharmacokinetics

Nitrates usually have good absorption from skin and gastrointestinal tract. Problem with oral administration is first pass effect. Hence for rapid action they are administered by sublingual route and the action starts within 1 minute. One more advantage with sublingual administration is that, in case of signs of overdose the tablet can be thrown out or can be swallowed. Swallowing will not produce the effect immediately and the magnitude of effect will also be less due to first pass effect.

Indications

Angina pectoris: Nitrates are used in all types of angina with different objectives. These are the drugs of choice in angina. In classical angina nitrates provide relief by reducing oxygen demand (due to vasodilatation) and by improving blood supply (due to coronary dilatation). In prinzmetal or variant angina nitrates relive coronary spasm and relieve pain. These agents are also used for prophylaxis of angina. Nitrates improve exercise tolerance in angina. β blockers and calcium channel blockers are combined with nitrates when monotherapy is not very effective in controlling angina.

Nitrates reduce workload of the heart and improve coronary circulation. They are drugs of choice in angina pectoris

Cardiac failure: By reducing preload, nitrates can reduce oxygen demand of the failing heart. Intravenous nitroglycerine is a drug of choice in cardiac failure.

MI: Immediate treatment of IV nitroglycerine in myocardial infarction can reduce the size of necrosis.

Nitrates are used in cardiovascular procedures to dilate coronary blood vessels.

Smooth muscle relaxation produced by nitrates is helpful in relieving spasms in gastrointestinal tract.

Cyanide poisoning: Nitrates convert hemoglobin into methemoglobin which combines with cyanide to form cyanomethemoglobin. Along with nitrates when Na thiosulfate is given, it breaks cyanomethemoglobin into methemoglobin and sodium thiocyanate, which are eliminated from body.

Figure 4.3 Mechanism of action of nitrates

Nitrates
↓
Denitration → Release of NO
↓
Reduced activation of guanylyl cyclase
↓
Increase in intracellular cyclic GMP (→ Reduces Ca influx in cells → Relaxation of blood vessels)
↓
Dephosphorylation of myosin light chain kinase
↓
Reduced activation of myosin
↓
Reduced actin-myosin coupling
↓
Reduced contraction of smooth muscles
↓
Relaxation of blood vessels

- Dilatation of veins (Major action) → ↓ Venous return → ↓ filling of heart ↓ Preload on heart → less energy is required to pump the blood i.e. ↓ oxygen demand for heart
- Dilation of large arteries (Minor action) → ↓ Peripheral resistance → ↓ afterload → Blood is pumped against less resistance → Decreased oxygen demand of heart
- Dilatation of coronaries → Mainly in large arteries → Favorable redistribution of blood in coronary arteries → Improvement in blood supply to heart.

Nitrates predominantly act on veins and coronaries and to some extent on larger arteries.

Adverse effects

Drop in BP, fainting, headache, flush are common side effects due to extension of pharmacological action. Blurred vision and dizziness also are sometimes observed. Reflex sympathetic stimulation produces palpitations. Methemoglobinemia is the side effect that can therapeutically be utilized in cyanide poisoning. Development of tolerance is another problem with nitrates, therefore intermittent discontinuation is required, especially for long acting nitrates. Sudden withdrawal of nitrates can cause spasms as withdrawal reaction. Tolerance is less with sublingual administration because body is not continuously exposed to the drug.

Headache is the commonest problem with nitrates.

Long term use of nitrates produces tolerance.

Nitroglycerine is the most commonly used nitrate.

Nitrates are used by various routes of administration.

Individual agents

Table 4.3 Nitrates

Individual agents	Features
Nitroglycerine	
Sublingual Nitroglycerine 0.3-0.6 mg	Relief within 1-2 minutes. Action lasts for half an hour. Treatment of choice in anginal attack
Nitroglycerine 0.4 mg aerosol	Immediate relief. Action for about 2 hours.
Oral sustained release nitroglycerine 2.5 - 15 mg	Relief is not rapid. May take an hour to start the action but action is maintained for about 8 hours.
Nitroglycerine ointment 15 mg/inch	Effective due to good cutaneous absorption.
Transdermal nitroglycerine patch 5 - 15 mg	Initiation of action takes 1 hours but action is maintained for 24 hours.
IV nitroglycerine 5 - 200 µg/min	For MI and cardiac failure.
Sublingual isosorbide dinitrate 2.5 - 10 mg oral isosorbide dinitrate 5 - 40 mg	Slow acting as compared to nitroglycerine.
Oral isosorbide mono nitrate 10-20 mg oral	Long acting. Without first pass effect. Metabolite of isosorbide dinitrate.
Erythrityl tetranitrate 30-60 mg oral	
Pentaerythritol tetranitrate 10-80 mg oral	Long acting. For prophylaxis.

Precautions and interactions

i) Nitrates produce hypotension if are taken along with other vasodilators or with alcohol.

ii) These agents reduce cardiac filling and are not used in hypovolemic conditions.

iii) Nitrates are used with caution in hepatic and renal impairment

iv) Dry mouth reduces absorption of sublingual nitrate.

Status

Nitrates are drugs of choice in all types of angina, for immediate relief and for prophylaxis. They are available by different routes. Their use in CCF and MI depends on the cardiovascular status. First pass metabolism and high chances of tolerance are the common problems.

CARDIAC GLYCOSIDES

Digitalis is a collective term that refers to a group of drugs that contains cardiac glycosides. Digitalis is originally obtained from foxglove plant. Different cardiac glycosides are digoxin, digitoxin, lanatoside, gitoxin, ouabain, etc.

Mechanism of action

Cardiac glycosides have two types of effects.

i) Direct effects, and

ii) Indirect effects

These effects may not be in the same direction. Some effects are opposite to each other.

Direct effects

Cell membrane of myocardial cell contains enzyme Na^+ K^+ ATPase. The enzyme hydrolyses ATP, sends Na^+ out of the cell and allows entry of K^+ inside the cells.

They improve contractions of heart and facilitate complete emptying of heart.

Cardiac glycosides inhibit activity of Na^+ K^+ ATPase. This inhibition increases Na^+ concentration, and reduces K^+ concentration inside the cell. This is followed by entry of calcium in the cell. Increase in intracellular concentration of Ca is responsible for increase contractibility of myocardial cells.

Indirect effects

1) Stimulation of vagus nerve,

2) Sensitization of SA node for acetylcholine, and

3) Sensitizations of baroreceptors.

All the actions mimic parasympathetic activity.

Heart rate is reduced by cardiac glycosides.

Combination of these two types of actions leads to:

1) Increased contractibility of heart

2) Complete emptying of ventricles, which improves ventricular ejection and cardiac output

3) Increased pumping: It improves perfusion which in turn reduces sympathetic overactivity. It subsequently reduces load on the heart.

4) Reduction in heart rate

5) Decreased generation and propagation of currents

6) Reduction in edema: cardiac glycosides, i) reduce sympathetic activity which improves renal blood flow and there is a diuretic action. ii) Improve pumping of blood and reduce back pressure of blood on veins. Both these actions reduce fluid overload and edema in CCF.

In brief, cardiac glycosides improve performance of heart without increasing consumption of oxygen and reduce edema. The actions are prominent in failing heart and not in normal heart.

Cardiac glycosides predominantly produce effects in failing heart.

Cardiac glycosides reduce edema associated with heart failure.

Pharmacokinetics

Cardiac glycosides are given by oral and intravenous routes. Oral route is a preferred route and intravenous drug is administered in case of emergency or severe vomiting. Absorption is reduced by food. Some amount is directly eliminated through kidneys and partly after metabolism by liver (proportion varies according to individual agent). Concentration in heart is much higher as compared to that in plasma. Cardiac glycosides are the drugs with very long half life.

Indications

Congestive cardiac failure

Cardiac glycosides offer following advantages in cardiac failure:

i) Improvement in contractile function
ii) Complete emptying
iii) Prolonged diastolic time
iv) Reduction in heart rate
v) Reduction in sympathetic overactivity
vi) Reduced edema

Cardiac glycosides improve performance of heart without increasing consumption of oxygen and reduce edema. They are especially useful in cardiac failure associated with arrhythmias and low output failure and not very effective in high output failure.

Cardiac glycosides are very effective in low output failure and in failure associated with arrhythmias.

Cardiac arrhythmia

Digitalis is used in atrial fibrillation, atrial flutter, especially when ventricular rate is rapid.

Toxicity

Digitalis toxicity is a crucial issue because it has narrow therapeutic range. Slight increase in the dose may alter effects and adverse effects to a large extent. Hypokalemia due to any cause increases digitalis toxicity.

Cardiac glycosides have narrow therapeutic range and severe toxic potential.

1) Cardiac toxicity: Digitalis causes extrasystole followed by AV dissociation or paroxysmal atrial tachycardia.

2) Depletion of intracellular potassium or increased in intracellular Ca are major consequences of digitalis therapy

3) CTZ (chemoreceptor trigger zone): Glycosides act on CTZ and produce visual disturbances, confusion, nausea, vomiting etc.

4) Adverse effects on GI tract: diarrhoea, abdominal pain, etc.

Hypokalemia due to any cause potentiates toxicity of cardiac glycosides

Due to all these adverse effects, proper precaution must be taken in elderly population, renal disorders, myocardial infraction and arrhythmia.

Interactions and precautions

Various adverse effects of digitalis demand lot of precautions:

i) Digitalis is contraindicated in AV block

ii) Drugs like quinidine, verapamil, indomethacin increase level of digoxin.

iii) Drugs like antacids, rifampicin, phenytoin reduce levels of digitalis.

iv) K sparing diuretics, corticosteroids induce hypokalemia and enhance digitalis toxicity.

Digitalis treatment demands lot of precautions.

Treatment of digitalis toxicity

Digoxin specific antibodies are administered in acute toxicity. If toxicity is manifested by ventricular arrhythmia, phenytoin (100 mg IV) is used. If it is manifested by bradycardia, atropine is the treatment of choice. Potassium is administered if AV block or hyperkalemia is not there.

Digitalization

As cardiac glycosides take a long time to achieve full effect, a loading dose is required to achieve full therapeutic effect. This is termed as digitalization. Digitalization can be done by oral and intravenous routes.

Digitalization is required for digitalis therapy.

Figure 4.4 Digitalization

Digitalization
- Oral
  - Slow digitalization → 0.25 mg digoxin/day → 1 Week → No response → 0.375 mg/day → 1 Week → No response → 0.5 mg/day
  - Rapid digitalization → 0.5 mg stat → 0.25 mg every 6 hr with close monitoring
- Intravenous → 0.25 - 1.0 mg

During first 24 hours maximum dose of digoxin should be 5 mg (oral) or 1 mg (IV) and oral maintenance dose should be up to 0.5 mg. Close monitoring over heart rate is required. It should not be less than 60 during the treatment.

Heart rate is monitored during digitalis treatment.

Individual agents

Table 4.4 Cardiac glycosides

Digoxin 0.125 - 0.5 mg	Fair oral absorption. Given by oral and IV route Metabolized less. Excreted unchanged in urine. Half-life 1-2 days Rapid onset: duration 1 week. Used for initiation and maintenance
Digitoxin 0.8-1.2 mg (loading) 0.05 - 0.2 mg maintenance	Maximum oral bioavailability: only by oral route Major part undergoes hepatic metabolism Used for maintenance therapy. Half-life: 5-7 days Slow onset. Duration 2-3 weeks.
Ouabain	Given only by IV route and is used only for emergency treatment.

Status of cardiac glycosides

Cardiac glycosides, now, are no more essential drugs for management of CCF. They are used in combination with diuretics and vasodilators and especially helpful in systolic dysfunction. Narrow therapeutic range and serious toxic manifestations are major limiting problems with these agents.

DIURETICS

These agents promote urine secretion. Diuretics increase amount of urine and reduce fluid overload of the body.

Classification of diuretics

Depending on the efficacy of promoting diuresis, they are classified as:

Figure 4.5 Diuretics

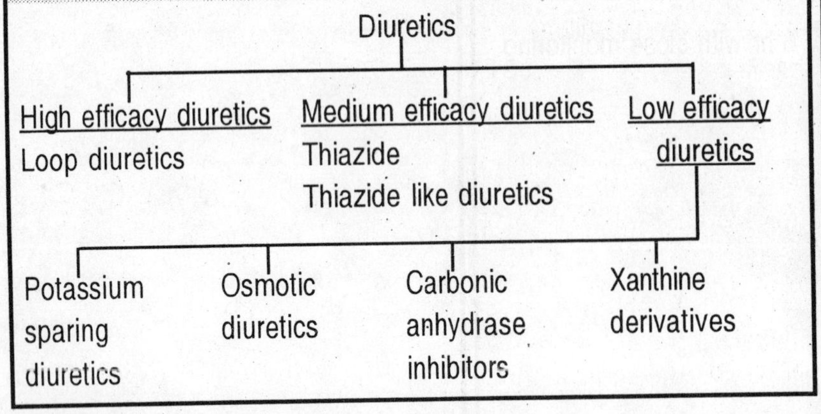

Physiological considerations

Nephron is a basic unit of kidney that forms the urine. Nephron has got following units (Refer figure 4.6): Bowman's capsule, proximal convoluted tubule, ascending and descending limb of loop of Henle and distal convoluted tubule. Distal convoluted tubule drains urine into collecting tubule. Collecting tubule drains urine into ureter. Cortex is outer part of kidney and medulla is inner portion.

Figure 4.6 Nephron

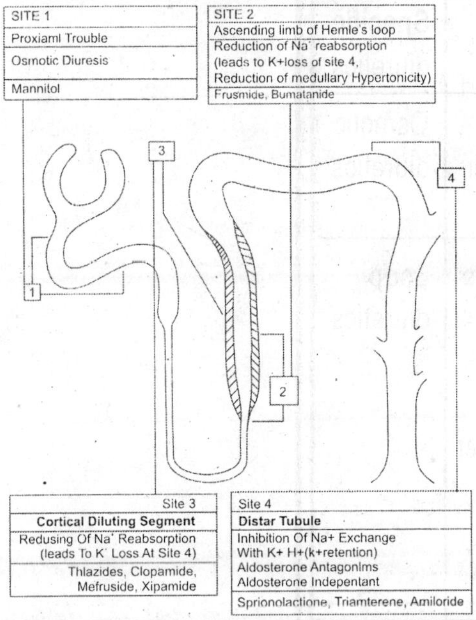

Three basic processes are involved in the formation of urine in nephron.

i) **Glomerular filtration:** It is filtration of blood and formation of urine in Bowman's capsule. About 180 L of urine is formed by this process.

ii) **Tubular reabsorption:** This is the process that reabsorbs a major fraction of urine back into the blood. Due to reabsorption, out of 180 L. formed urine, excretion is only that of 1.5-2 liters.

iii) **Tubular secretion:** Some contents are actively transported from blood into urine.

Kidneys function on the principle of osmosis

To understand the mechanism of action of diuretics, it is essential to recollect the concept of osmosis. If there are two compartments that are separated by semipermeable membrane and they contain different concentration of solutions; there is a natural tendency to make concentrations in both compartments equal. Fluids and electrolytes move in the direction that will make concentrations on both sides equal.

Similarly, if some electrolytes (like Na or K) are more in urine, water from body is pulled into urine. If electrolytes are reabsorbed out of urine in blood, some fluid in urine also goes with electrolytes. Thus, fluid and electrolytes together decide the amount of urine.

Table 4.5 indicates physiological actions that take place at different sites in nephron and how these actions are altered by different diuretics.

Table 4.5 Actions of diuretics			
Site	**Physiological function**	**Alterations by diuretics**	**Specific** diuretics
I Proximal tubule (cortex)	Reabsorption of urine, that is formed by glomerular filtration	Diuretics prevent reabsorption of water and Na	Osmotic diuretics
II Ascending Loop (medulla)	Chlorides are actively transported from tubules back to interstitial fluid. They carry Na with them. Water is not accompanied, as this part is not permeable for water	Diuretics block active transport of chloride and so Na from the tubules. Keep electrolytes and water in tubules.	Loop diuretics
III Ascending loop. (cortex)	Rapid active transport of Na and chlorides out of loop into extracellular fluid.	Diuretics prevent Na reabsorption & maintain Na in urine. Therefore water is also not reabsorbed	Thiazide diuretics
IV Distal tubules (cortex)	Exchange of Na from urine with K from the interstitial fluid.	Diuretics prevent exchange of Na and K. So Na remains in urine and K^+ and H^+ are retained in body	Potassium sparing diuretics

High efficacy diuretics or loop diuretics

These drugs are highly effective agents. They increase the amount of urine to a large extent and are called as high ceiling diuretics. Ex. frusemide (furosemide), bumetanide, piretanide, ethacrynic acid etc.

Mechanism of action: These agents act at site II (Figure 4.6 ascending loop of Henle in medulla). They prevent active transport of Na and chloride out of tubules. Therefore electrolyte concentration of urine is maintained and water loss in further segments is prevented.

Additional actions that promote diuresis

i) Weak carbonic anhydrase inhibitory action

ii) Increase in calcium and magnesium secretion

iii) Dilatation of renal and peripheral blood vessels

iv) Increase in potassium, water and phosphate excretion

Loop diuretics act at ascending loop and block active reabsorption of Na and chlorides.

Thus these agents increase quantity of chlorides and Na in urine. Dilatation of arteries by these diuretics reduces after load and that of veins reduces preload. It helps in reducing edema.

Pharmacokinetics

These drugs can be given by oral, IM or IV route. Absorption by oral route though is rapid, bioavailability is not very high. Bioavailability is further reduced in CCF. These drugs are excreted in urine and bile.

Loop diuretics act on blood vessels, reduce preload, afterload and edema.

Indications

Systemic and pulmonary edema: These agents are highly effective in reducing edema of all types - cardiac, hepatic and renal. Depending on emergency, oral or intravenous route is selected. Immediate relief is obtained in pulmonary edema by vasodilatation (reduced preload on heart and lungs) and subsequent effects are due to reduced fluid and electrolyte overload.

Cerebral edema: Though these agents can reduce cerebral edema, they are rarely used for this indication.

Loop diuretics are used in systemic and pulmonary edema.

Hypertension: Thiazides are the preferred diuretics in hypertension but only in resistant cases or if immediate relief is required.

Miscellaneous indications

i) These drugs are used to induce forced diuresis in barbiturate poisoning. They promote elimination of barbiturates.

ii) Calcium excretion caused by these drugs is therapeutically utilized in calcium stones.

Adverse effects

Majority of side effects are related to pharmacological actions. Excess Na loss in urine leads to reduced Na content in blood: hyponatremia. Similarly there is hypocalcemia and hypomagnesemia.

Hypokalemia - These agents prevent Na reabsorption at site II. This retained excess Na at site II when reaches at site III, it pulls large amount of K in tubules and there is loss of K from body, which leads to hypokalemia. Hypotension, nausea, vomiting, hearing loss, pancreatitis, raised urates are some additional side effects of loop diuretics.

Adverse effects of loop diuretics are predominantly due to extension of pharmacological actions.

Precaution and interactions:

i) These agents produce hypokalemia and increase chances of toxicity of cardiac glycosides.

ii) Potassium supplements or potassium sparing diuretics are added in case of severe hypokalemia.

iii) These agents interfere in antidiabetic effect of oral hypoglycemics.

iv) They interfere in metabolism and excretion of OC pills, steroids and NSAIDs.

v) These drugs are used with caution in hepatic and renal disorders.

Hypokalemia is associated with loop diuretics.

Individual agents	Features
Frusemide oral 20-80 mg IV 10-80 mg max 200 mg	A drug of choice. Oral action starts within 1 hour and lasts for 6 hours, IV or IM action starts within up to 5 minutes and lasts for 2-3 hours.
Bumetanide 1-5 mg oral 0.5-4 mg IV max- 15 mg	More potent agent. Preferred in patients who are resistant to frusemide. Better bioavailability.
Ethacrynic acid 50-150 mg	More potent but side effects are more. Used in severe and resistant cases.

Table 4.6 Loop diuretics

Resistance to loop diuretics

Delayed absorption (due to congestion of GI mucosa) or inability to reach at the site of action (due to reduced renal blood flow) can lead to failure of action of loop diuretics. This is termed as resistance to loop diuretics.

Loop diuretics are used to initiate the therapy and maintenance is usually done with medium efficacy diuretics.

Status: Loop diuretics are drugs of choice when rapid immobilization of fluids is required. They are used to initiate the therapy and maintenance is usually done with medium efficacy diuretics. Adverse effects are mainly extension of pharmacological action.

Thiazide and related diuretics

These are the most commonly used diuretics. They have moderate efficacy. The agents include chlorthiazide, polythiazide, hydrochlorthiazide, bendroflumethiazide. Some drugs by structure are not thiazides but act like them and are called as thiazide like diuretics. They include chlorthalidone, metolazone, xipamide, indapamide, etc.

Thiazides are most widely used diuretics.

Mechanism of action: (Refer table 4.5)

These agents act in the cortex, at ascending loop of Henle. Prevention of reabsorption of Na, and keeping Na and water in urine is the major mechanism of action. Additionally these agents have some CA inhibitor action. They also reduce GFR. (Glomerular filtration rate) by their action on blood vessels.

Non-renal actions

1) Thiazides reduce responsiveness of blood vessels to Noradrenaline

2) They have direct relaxing action on blood vessels. Both these non renal actions contribute to the antihypertensive effects of thiazides. There is a gradual fall in BP

3) Thiazides reduce insulin release.

Non-renal actions of thiazides are important for reduction in blood pressure.

Pharmacokinetics

They are administered orally and action starts within an hour. All agents have more or less same actions. The difference is mainly in the duration of action. Longer acting agents have high lipid solubility and more protein binding.

Indications

Mild to moderate edema: These agents reduce fluid overload and reduce edema. They are mainly useful in edema of cardiac origin.

Hypertension: Thiazides are used as first line agents in management of hypertension. They produce effects gradually. Antihypertensive effects are due to renal and non renal actions.

Diuretics: Paradoxically, these agents reduce volume of urine in diabetes insipidus (reduced secretion of antidiuretic hormone).

Adverse effects

Hypokalemia is a common side effect. The reason for it is very much similar to that in loop diuretics (Refer Page 153) but magnitude is more. So these agents are used with potassium sparing diuretics. Additional side effects are agranulocytosis, GI upset, impotence, rashes, hyperuricemia, increased low density lipoproteins (harmful lipids), etc.

Thiazides are used in edema and hypertension.

Interactions and precautions

1) Hypokalemia induced by these agents increases the toxicity of cardiac glycosides.

2) Long term administration of thiazides suppresses secretion of insulin.

3) They are used with caution in hepatic and renal failure.

Thiazides induce loss of K and are used with potassium sparing diuretics.

Table 4.7 Thiazides

Individual agents and dose	Features
Chlorthiazide 125-500 mg	A classical thiazide Duration 6-12 hours
Hydrochlorothiazide 12.5-200 mg	Long acting. Used in calcium stones and diabetes insipidus.
Bendroflumethiazide 2.5 to 10 mg	A classical thiazide
Indapamide 2.5 to 5 mg	Thiazide like diuetics. Less side effects on lipid profile. Preferred in hypertension. Potency same. Longer duration of action.
Metolazone 2.5-20 mg	Thiazide like diuetics Additional action on proximal tubules
Xipamide 20-60 mg	Thiazide like diuetics Longer duration. Preferred in diabetes
Chlorthalidone 12.5 - 200 mg	Duration up to 72 hours. Used for diabetes insipidus.

Status

This is the most widely used class of diuretics. They are used for first line management of hypertension. These agents can be combined with other antihypertensives. Mild to moderate edema, especially of cardiac origin, responds well to thiazides. Potassium loss is a major problem with thiazides, so they are combined with potassium sparing diuretics. Non renal actions contribute in antihypertensive effects.

Potassium sparing diuretics

As the name suggests these agents (i) promote diuresis but (ii) reduce potassium loss in urine that is usually associated with other diuretics. These agents are classified into 2 groups.

i) Aldosterone antagonist: Spironolactone

ii) Directly acting on channels: Triamterene, Amiloride.

Mechanism of action: These agents act at site IV: distal tubules in cortex.

1) Mechanism of action of spironolactone:

Aldosterone is a corticosteroid in body that promotes renal reabsorption of Na and excretion of potassium. Spironolactone, in distal tubule, blocks the receptors of aldosterone and prevents reabsorption of Na and excretion of K. Reduced Na reabsorption facilitates diuresis while prevention of K excretion reduces loss of potassium. It also has some antihypertensive actions like thiazide and some direct action that stimulates excretion of calcium.

Potassium sparing diuretics reduce loss of K in urine.

2) Mechanism of amiloride and triamterene:

These agents directly act on Na channel in the distal tubules and prevent reabsorption of Na. This also prevents secretion of K into tubules. These agents do not act on aldosterone receptors.

Indications

These agents are used in edema and hypertension but usually not used alone. They are used in combination with loop diuretics or thiazide diuretics to support the diuretic action and to compensate loss of potassium.

Spironolactone, due to its blocking action on aldosterone receptors, is used in primary hypersecretion of aldosterone.

Potassium sparing diuretics are used in combination with thiazides or loop diuretics.

Adverse effects

Reduced excretion of K in urine increases its concentration in blood. Thus hyperkalemia can be a major problem with these drugs, especially if K supplementations are provided to patients. GI disturbances, headache, cramps are some additional problems. Spironolactone itself is a steroid and can cause side effects like gynecomastia, menstrual irregularities, sexual disturbances, mental confusion, etc.

Spironolactone is effective in presence of overactivity of aldosterone.

Precautions and interactions

i) Potassium supplements are not given along with these drugs.

iii) These drugs are used with caution in elderly population.

Table 4.8 Potassium sparing diuretics

Individual agents and doses	Features
Spironolactone 50-200 mg/day Oral	Steroid. Causes hormone related side effects. Mainly effective in presence of excess aldosterone. Its active metabolite is canrenone.
Triamterene 100-200 mg/day Oral	No action on aldosterone receptors. Effective even when aldosterone activity is less. Onset delayed but action is long term. Steroidal side effects are not present
Amiloride 5-10 mg/day Oral	Similar to triamterene and more potent. Early onset and short duration.

Status: These are weak diuretics and are not used alone. They are commonly used in combination with thiazide or loop diuretics.

Osmotic diuretics

Mannitol is the commonly used agent from this class. It is a pharmacologically inactive substance with low molecular weight and is a weak diuretic. Urea and glucose also act as osmotic diuretics.

Mechanism of action

Mannitol acts at site I (Refer figure 4.5) on proximal tubules in cortex. The drug, along with the urine, is filtered by glomerulus but is not reabsorbed from the tubule. Being osmotically active, it increases osmolarity and so volume of urine. It predominantly maintains water in urine and less sodium is excreted. Additionally it also prevents Na and water reabsorption in loop of Henle. Increase in renal blood flow is also reported with it.

Pharmacokinetics

The drug is not absorbed orally and is given only by IV route

Indication

Mannitol is not used to reduce circulatory edema. It is used mainly to reduce risky localized edema.

1) Threatened renal failure is associated with hypotension and hypovolemia, where GFR is markedly reduced. Mannitol maintains GFR and urine flow in these situations. Other diuretics are usually not effective.

2) Raised Intracranial pressure or cerebral edema can be treated with IV mannitol.

3) Mannitol reduces intraocular pressure in congestive glaucoma and provides pain relief (Refer page 104).

Osmotic diuretics are mainly used to reduce dangerous localized edema and not circulatory edema.

Osmotic diuretics reduce intraocular and intracranial pressure.

Osmotic diuretics improve glomerular filtration and maintain flow of urine

4) Mannitol is used to induce forced diuresis in barbiturate poisoning.

Adverse effects

Headache, nausea, cellular dehydration, GI disturbances and hypersensitivity are common side effects.

Precautions:

Leakage of mannitol from site of infusion causes skin reactions.

Mannitol is not suitable for reducing edema caused by circulatory failure because it expands body volume.

It causes extra strain on impaired heart and produce pulmonary edema.

It is not used when there is cardiac failure, pulmonary edema and when renal failure is established.

Dosage: 10-20% solution of IV mannitol is effective for rapid relief.

Status: Mannitol is mainly used to reduce intracranial and intraocular pressure and to maintain glomerular filtration.

Carbonic anhydrase inhibitors (CAI)

Though these agents are discussed under title diuretics, they are no more used as diuretics. They have very weak diuretic action. Agents from this class are acetazolamide, dichlorphenamide and ethoxzolamide

Mechanism of action

Carbonic anhydrase (CA) is an enzyme present in kidney, stomach, eye, brain, RBCs, etc. It is involved in following reaction.

$$CO_2 + H_2O \underset{\uparrow}{\rightleftharpoons} H_2CO_3 \rightleftharpoons H^+ + HCO_3^-$$

Carbonic anhydrase

In kidneys, enzyme carbonic anhydrase makes H^+ available, which is exchanged with Na in the tubules. CAIs inhibit CA and reduces formation of H^+ and HCO_3^-. When H^+ is not available for exchange, Na reabsorption is reduced and diuresis is promoted. HCO_3^- is essential for formation of aqueous humor in eye. CAIs limit availability of HCO_3^- and reduce formation of aqueous humor. In similar way it reduces formation of CSF in brain.

CIAs are not used as diuretics. They are used in glaucoma and mountain sickness.

Indications

Glaucoma: It is the condition characterized by increased intraocular pressure (Refer page 103). CAIs reduce formation of aqueous humor (by limiting HCO_3^-) and reduce intraocular pressure.

Prophylaxis of mountain sickness: Mountain sickness is disease of high altitude (rapid climb above 3000 m) and is characterized by nausea, lassitude, headache, impaired judgement, pulmonary and cerebral edema. These symptoms are proposed to be due to alkalosis at high altitude. CAIs induce acidosis, improve respiratory drive and maintain oxygen tension in blood. They cannot control cerebral and pulmonary edema.

CAIs are also used as adjuvants in epileptic disorders and for alkalinization of urine (alkalinization of urine increases elimination of acidic drugs)

Side effects: Drowsiness, fever, rash, hypokalemia, hypersensitivity, acidosis are some of the side effects of CAIs.

Dose: Acetazolamide is the commonly used drug and is given in dose of 250 mg OD or BD

Status: CAIs are not used as diuretics. They are used for mountain sickness and glaucoma.

VASODILATORS

This is a collective term used for drugs, which dilate blood vessels. These agents are classified as follows:

Figure 4.7 Vasodilators

Vasodilators

Venodilators	Arterial dilators	Acting on both veins and arteries
Nitrates	Calcium channel blockers	ACE inhibitors
	Potassium channel openers	A II antagonists
	Directly acting agents	α blockers
		Nitroprusside

Most of these agents are already discussed in previous sections. Some miscellaneous agents are discussed below.

Hydralazine

It is a directly acting arterial dilator with almost no action on veins.

Mechanism of action

Hydralazine generates nitric oxide (NO) in arterial walls and stimulates production of cyclic GMP and produces arterioler dilatation. (Refer page 145). Arterial dilatation leads to decreased peripheral resistance and fall in BP. This produces reflex sympathetic activation and heart rate and cardiac output is increased and fluids are retained. Cerebral, coronary and renal blood flow is increased by this agent.

Hydralazine is directly acting arteriolar dilator

Pharmacokinetics

The drug is well absorbed orally, undergoes first pass effect, metabolized in liver and excreted by kidney. Though half-life of drug is short its binding to vascular cells prolongs the duration of action. It produces effects slowly.

Indications

Hydralazine is used as a second line drug in the management of hypertension and usually given along with β blockers. It is also used in CCF along with nitrates. Hydralazine is avoided in myocardial infarction and angina as it can produce reflex sympathetic stimulation.

Hydralazine is avoided in MI and angina.

Adverse effects

These include flushing, throbbing headache and nasal congestion (all are due to vasodilatation), palpitation (due to reflex sympathetic stimulation). To avoid these, β blockers are administered together. Drowsiness, systemic lupus erythematous syndrome, fever, arthritis like condition, etc. are additional side effects. GI side effects are nausea, vomiting and acidity. Dose - 50-300 mg oral, 5-10 mg IV over 20 minutes

Hydralazine is used as second line drug in hypertension and is given along with β blockers.

Potassium channel openers

These agents dilate arteries through their action on K channels and are used in variety of cardiac and some noncardiac disorders. Ex. Minoxidil, diazoxide, nicorandil.

Mechanism

These drugs activate ATP dependent potassium channel and opening of these channels allows outflow of K ions resulting in repolarization and relaxation of smooth muscles. Thus, these agents produce arterial dilatation and relaxation of some visceral muscles.

Indications: Indications vary according to individual agents. They are discussed in the table 4.9.

Diazoxide, minoxidil and nicorandil are potassium channel openers.

Table 4.9 Potassium channel openers

Individual agents and doses	Features
Diazoxide 1-3 mg/kg max 150 mg IV	Arterial dilator and is used in emergencies for rapid reduction in BP. Effect is obtained within 5 minutes. It inhibits release of insulin from pancreas and is used in insulinoma. Hyperglycemia, hyperuricemia are side effects. Reflex sympathetic stimulation is common.
Minoxidil 2% topical lotion or spray 5-50 mg/day Oral	Arterial dilator. Highly potent but toxic. Reflex sympathetic activity produces tachycardia, palpitation etc. Rarely used for hypertension. Improvement in cutaneous blood flow and increased hair growth are the side effects. Therefore minoxidil is effectively used in alopecia for hair growth. It improves microcirculation around hair follicle and also directly stimulates hair follicle.
Nicorandil 5-20 mg BD	Added effect on veins and coronary blood vessels. Effective in angina.

Diazoxide is used only in hypertensive emergencies and is administered only by IV route.

Nitroprusside

It is a vasodilator that acts on both veins and arteries and is used in hypertensive emergencies.

Mechanism of action

Spliting of nitroprusside produces NO (nitric oxide) and relaxes smooth muscles of both arteries and veins. (Refer page 145). This reduces preload and afterload. Reduction in PR reduces BP rapidly. Action starts within a second and has very short duration- up to 5 minutes. Cardiac output is also reduced due to decreased venous return.

Nitroprusside dilates veins and arteries

Nitroprusside is used in hypertensive emergency.

Indications

Hypertensive emergency 0.1 - 0.3 mg/min IV

CCF: Nitroprusside, by reducing preload and afterload, reduces oxygen demand. It can also be used in myocardial infarction.

Adverse effects

These include palpitations, weakness and vomiting. Long term infusion leads to psychoses.

COAGULATION

Physiological considerations

Coagulation of blood is a sequential process by which multiple coagulation factors of blood interact resulting in formation of an insoluble clot. The system works by two modes. Extrinsic system is activated in response to tissue damage and is a rapid acting system while intrinsic system is slow and works in response to vascular damage. There are total 12 clotting factors involved in the process of coagulation.

Figure 4.8 Coagulation system and fibrinolytic system

Extrinsic system → Cascade of factors → Factor X → Activated factor (Xa)

Intrinsic system → Cascade of factors → Factor X → Activated factor (Xa)

Activated factor (Xa) ↓

Prothrombin (II) → Thrombin

Thrombin ↓

Fibrinogen → Fibrin (soluble)

↓

Fibrin (non soluble)

↓

Formation of clot

↓

Breaking of clot

↓

Fibrin degradation products

Fibrinolytic system

↓

Plasminogen → Plasmin → ↓ (Breaking of clot)

↑

Factor XII and tPA

Fibrinolytic system is the continuation of clotting system and it is involved in breaking down the clot. Factor XII and tpA activates plasminogen into plasmin, which breaks the clot. Drugs can alter both clotting system and fibrinolytic system. Drugs either activate or inhibit coagulation system or fibrinolytic system. Depending on that drugs are termed as coagulants, anticoagulants, fibrinolytics and antifibrinolytics.

Anticoagulants

Drugs can activate or inactivate coagulation process or fibrinolytic system.

Anticoagulants prevent process of clotting but do not break a clot that is already formed. **In-vitro anticoagulants:** These agents are added in blood that is withdrawn for pathological tests. They prevent clotting of blood when blood is outside the body. **In-vivo anticoagulants:** These agents are administered in the body and they prevent clotting inside the body.

Anticoagulants do not break thrombus: they prevent formation of it.

Figure 4.9 Anticoagulants

- Anticoagulants
  - In vitro
    - Heparin
    - Sodium citrate
    - Sodium oxalate
    - Sodium edetate
  - In vivo
    - Injectable
      - Heparin
      - Heparinoids
        - ↓
        - Ancrod
        - Dextran
    - Oral
      - Coumarin
        - Warfarin
        - Bishydroxycoumarin
        - Acenocoumarin
      - Indandione
        - Phenindione

HEPARIN

It is a naturally occurring substance in mast cells and it is mainly present in lungs and liver. For therapeutic purpose it is obtained from animals like pigs and ox. Molecular weight of heparin ranges from 3,000 to 30,000 with an average of 15000.

Mechanism of action

Antithrombin III is a substance in the body that inhibits prothrombin and activated factor X (Xa). Heparin, in very low doses, increases the activity of antithrombin III and potentiates inhibition of two clotting factors. This results in prevention of clotting process. In high doses heparin inhibits clotting factor IX and X.

Some additional actions of Heparin:

i) Heparin inhibits platelet aggregation and helps in preventing clot formation.

ii) It reduces proliferation of vascular smooth muscles.

iii) Heparin has got some antiinflammatory action.

Heparin acts by increasing activity of antithrombin. It is rapid acting anticoagulant.

Pharmacokinetics

IM administration of heparin causes hematoma. Heparin is poorly absorbed from GI tract and therefore is often administered by IV or SC routes. It follows both zero order and first order kinetics. It is predominantly distributed in mast cells; which acts as store of external heparin. As it does not cross placental barrier, it can safely be given during pregnancy.

Indication and contraindications

(Refer indications of anticoagulants on page 164).

Adverse effects

Bleeding, hematuria, thrombocytopenia, alopecia, osteoporosis and hypersensitivity reactions.

Dosing

Heparin is measured in international units 1 IU is the amount that prevents 1 ml of citrated sheep plasma from clotting for 1 hour after addition of 0.2 ml of 1% $CaCl_2$ solution.
1 mg = 120-140 U activity.

Heparin is administered by IV or SC route.

Heparin is safe in pregnancy and lactation.

Prophylactic dose of heparin to prevent thromboembolism is 5000 U SC BD (started before operation and continued till discharge)
Therapeutic dose to prevent extension of thrombus:
10,000 U/hr SC or IV. In children 50-100 U/kg
Infusion - 5000 U followed by 20,000 U/day

Low molecular weight heparin

These molecules are obtained from depolymerization of standard heparin. Molecular weight ranges from 1,000 to 9,000. Their major action is on Xa and comparatively less action is on prothrombin.

Advantages

i) Higher bioavailability,
ii) Long half-life, longer duration of action, therefore once a day administration,
iii) More predictable clinical response,
iv) Reduced chances of hemorrhagic complications.
Ex. Enoxaparin, Dalteparin, Finzaparin are the agents that are used in almost all the indications where heparin is used.

Low molecular weight heparins offer several advantages over standard heparin.

Oral anticoagulants

These are agents, which prevent clotting and unlike heparin can be given orally. They do not have in vitro activity.

Figure 4.10 Mechanism of action of oral anticoagulants

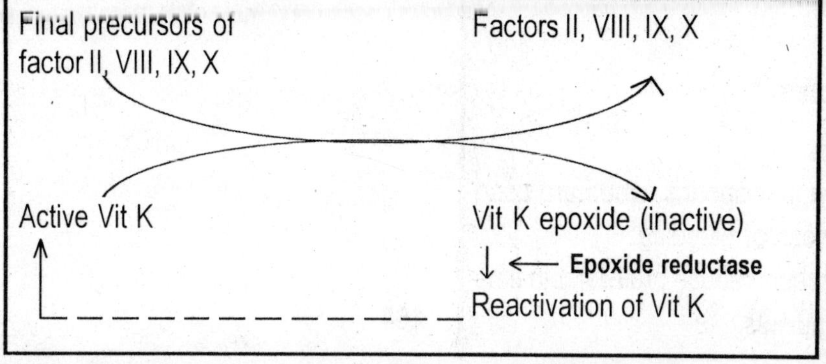

Final step in synthesis of clotting factor II ,VIII, IX, X requires active Vit K. Active form of Vit K itself gets converted into Vit K epoxide which is an inactive form. Enzyme epoxide reductase again converts it into active form and Vit K is available for synthesis of clotting factors. (Refer figure 4.10).

Oral anticoagulants are structurally similar to Vit K and act as substrate for enzyme epoxide reductase. Thus, Vit K epoxide or inactive Vit K is not converted into active Vit K and is not made available for synthesis of clotting factors. These agents prevent synthesis of clotting factors and do not have any action on clotting factors that are already formed. Therefore the initiation of action is slow, but action is prolonged. Genetic resistance to warfarin is reported in few individuals.

Oral anticoagulants prevent synthesis of clotting factors and do not have any action on clotting factors that are already formed.

Pharmacokinetics

Warfarin is a prototype agent that is used most commonly. It is a mixture of two isomers R and S, out of which S is more potent. These drugs are well absorbed orally. They are highly protein bound. They cross placenta and are secreted in milk. Their action is not rapid but lasts for 1 week.

Adverse effects

Bleeding is a major adverse effect. Common bleeding sites are gastrointestinal tract, renal and cerebral vessels. Cutaneous reactions, skin necrosis are additional problems with oral anticoagulants. Effects and adverse effects are exaggerated in Vit K deficiency, liver disorder and malnutrition because in these disorders formation of clotting factors is already hampered.

Contraindications to anticoagulants: (both heparin and oral anticoagulants)

1) Situations in which there are chances of bleeding: like piles, peptic ulcers, malignancies, thrombocytopenia, hypertension etc. (anticoagulants may increase chances of bleeding in these situations).

2) Hepatic or renal failure,

3) Subacute bacterial endocarditis: (anticoagulants may increase chances of emboli),

4) Critical surgeries like neurosurgeries,

5) Pregnancy : Oral anticoagulants (especially warfarin) produce growth retardation, hypoplastic bones, fetal hemorrhage, CNS defects and death. But heparin can safely be given during pregnancy.

Oral anticoagulants take around 3 days to achieve full effect.

Bleeding due to anticoagulants is treated by

i) Withdrawal of the drug,

ii) Blood transfusion,

iii) Administration of Vit K and clotting factors.

Drug interactions of oral anticoagulants

1) NSAIDs, heparin, anabolic steroids, cephalosporins, when are used along with anticoagulants, increase chances of bleeding.

2) Barbiturates, griseofulvin and carbamazepin reduce prothrombin time and interfere in the action of oral anticoagulants.

Indications for anticoagulants (both heparin and oral)

Anticoagulants do not break thrombus that is formed but they prevent formation of thrombus and inhibit extension of existing thrombus. Usually heparin is used to initiate the treatment for short prevention and oral anticoagulants for maintenance. Following are the indications:

1) To prevent formation of thrombus in high risk situations like:
i) Atrial fibrillation.
ii) Prosthetic heart valves
iv) Elderly population
v) Bed-ridden patients
vi) Fractures.

2) Myocardial infarction
IV infusion or high dose subcutaneous administration of heparin (12,500 units) reduces mortality in patients of MI. Otherwise 5,000 units BD is also effective to prevent thrombosis till patient becomes ambulatory. It is continued with the treatment of warfarin for next 3-6 months. In unstable angina anticoagulants are used along with aspirin to prevent MI.

3) Prophylaxis (prior to surgery): In cardiac, retinal or vascular surgeries anticoagulant treatment is started 2 hours before surgeries and continued till discharge. Heparin is a preferred agent for this.

4) To prevent extension of established thrombus.

5) To prevent pulmonary embolism.

6) Along with thrombolytic therapy, these agents are administered to prevent formation of new thrombus.

7) Anticoagulants are also used to prevent stroke due to atrial fibrillation.

Individual agents are discussed in table 4.10 on page 166.

Status

These drugs are used to prevent formation and extension of thrombus. Therapy is usually initiated with heparin and continued with oral anticoagulants. Recently, in many conditions, due to adverse effects and contraindication, the role of anticoagulants is becoming controversial, especially when compared to antiplatelet agents.

Anticoagulant therapy is usually initiated with heparin and continued with oral anticoagulants.

Table 4.10 Anticoagulants

Individual agents and dose	Features
Heparin	Only injectable administration. Action starts immediately. Can be given in early pregnancy but not in later stages. Short duration: up to 6 hrs. Used for initiation of therapy or for short prevention.
Warfarin 10 mg OD for 2 days then dose adjusted according to PT from 2 - 5 mg	Orally administered Drug of choice among oral anticoagulants Comparatively slow action. Takes up to 3 days to reach full therapeutic action. Used for maintenance of therapy. Not used in pregnancy. Duration of action up to one week.
Acenocoumarin Loading 8-12 mg Maintenance 2-8 mg	Almost similar profile to warfarin but duration of action is little short and GI disturbances are more common. Rarely used drugs
Bishydroxycoumarin Loading dose: 200 mg Maintenance dose: 50-100 mg	Profile similar to warfarin except longer duration and more GI side effects.
Phenidiones	Due to serious hemorrhagic side effects, agranulocytosis, edema, hepatic and renal damage, etc., these drugs should not be used. Or used only in coumarin intolerance.

Warfarin is most commonly used oral anticoagulant.

Dose of warfarin is adjusted according to PT (Prothrombin Time)

Anticoagulant treatment is usually initiated with heparin and maintained with oral anticoagulants.

FIBRINOLYTIC AGENTS

Fibrinolytic agents break thrombus that is already formed and reestablish the circulation. They are also called as thrombolytic agents.

Figure 4.11 Fibrinolytic agents

Fibrinolytic agents

- Therapeutic agents
  - ↓ Streptokinase, Urokinase, Alteplase (rt-PA)
- Naturally occuring in the body
  - ↓ t-PA, Kallikrein

Fibrinolytic agents break a clot that is already formed and re-establish circulation.

Mechanism of action

These agents act on fibrinolytic system (Refer page 161).

Figure 4.12 Mechanism of action of fibrinolytics

Plasminogen
↓ ← Fibrinolytic agents activate plasminogen.
Plasmin (fibrinolysin)
↓
Destruction of fibrin
↓
Breakdown of clot

Indications

Myocardial Infarction (MI)

These drugs are used as first line drugs in MI. Ideally best results are achieved in first 3 hours but they can be given up to 12 hours. Recanalization of vessel is the basic objective of the treatment. The treatment with anticoagulant drugs is initiated immediately after giving thrombolytic agents.

Fibrinolytic agents are drugs of choice in MI.

Ideally best results are achieved in first 3 hours but they can be given up to 12 hours.

Deep vein thrombosis

Fibrinolytic agents are not routinely indicated; but when there is massive emboli formation, fibrinolytic therapy is used.

Pulmonary embolism

In patients, not prone for bleeding, in massive embolism, these drugs are administered. But their role is controversial.

These drugs are used in patients who have massive embolism but are not prone for bleeding

Miscellaneous indications

Ocular thrombosis, thrombosed arteriovenous shunt, arterial occlusion.

Table 4.11 Fibrinolytics

Individual agents and dose	Features
Streptokinase (1.5 million U IV over 1 hour)	Obtained from β hemolytic streptococci. Comparatively cheaper but side effects are more.
Urokinase (7.5 lac U over 1 hr)	Obtained from cultures of fetal kidney cells. Comparatively lesser side effects.
Alteplase (rt PA) 10 mg IV bolus 50 mg over 1 hour 40 mg over next 2 hr	Obtained by recombinant genetic technology. It does not act on all plasminogen in the body but on the plasminogen that is attached to thrombus. Hence, higher thrombolytic activity and less adverse effects are produced.
Antistreptase	Longer acting agent.

rt-PA has selective action on the plasmin that is attached to clot. This increases the effectivity and reduces side effects.

Adverse effects

Fibrinolytic action of these agents is systemic and not selective. Therefore they reduce overall clotting ability of blood. It leads to bleeding, which is the most significant adverse effect associated with fibrinolytic agents. Therefore these agents are avoided in bleeding disorders, trauma, recent surgeries, peptic ulcer and hypertension. Arrhythmia, allergic reactions, fever are some additional adverse effects. These drugs are not used during pregnancies.

Status

Fibrinolytic agents are used as first line agents in MI. But treatment must be initiated before 12 hours (best before 3 hrs.) Bleeding disorder is common adverse effect. They are also effectively used in breaking venous thrombi and emboli.

Fibrinolytic agents are contraindicated in bleeding disorders, recent surgeries, peptic ulcer, pregnancy, hypertension, etc.

ANTIPLATELET AGENTS

Process of clotting starts with adhesion of platelets to vessel wall. Adhesion, then is responsible for platelet aggregation. Antiplatelet agents interfere in platelet function. They prevent aggregation of platelets. Ex. Aspirin, dipyridamole, ticlopidine, sufinpyrazone and epoprostol.

Mechanism of action

Aspirin: Cylcooxygenase is an enzyme required for synthesis of thromboxane. Thromboxane stimulates platelet aggregation. Aspirin inhibits enzyme cyclooxygenase and prevent formation of thromboxane. 75-150 mg/day is the dose of aspirin required for prevention of platelet aggregation. It is avoided in acid peptic disorder and bronchospasm.

Dipyridamole: It prevents degradation and uptake of adenosine. It makes more adenosine available at the site. Adenosine causes vasodilatation and reduces platelet aggregation. It also increases cyclic AMP. Increased cyclic AMP produces PGI and inhibit platelet aggregation. Dipyridamole additionally inhibits enzyme phosphodiesterase, which is involved in metabolism of cyclic AMP. Inhibition of this enzymes results in accumulation of cAMP. (Dose: 75-300 mg/day oral).

Antiplatelet agents inhibit aggregation of platelets and prevent formation of clot.

Ticlopidine: It directly interacts with platelets and inhibits binding of fibrinogen to platelets, which prevents formation of clot. Dose 250 mg BD oral.

Epoprostol: It is a prostaglandin that directly prevents platelet aggregation.

Indications for antiplatelet agents

1) Myocardial infarction : These agents are used immediately after MI to reduce extension of the clot and also used for prophylaxis i.e. to prevent formation of clots.

2) Transient ischemic attacks: It is the common complication in cerebrovascular disorders and is prevented by antiplatelet agents.

3) During coronary implants, prosthetic surgeries and arterial grafts

chances of thrombus formation are exaggerated. These are prevented by antiplatelet agents. They are usually used along with anticogulants.
4) These agents prevent thrombus formation in peripheral vascular disorders.

Pentoxyphylline

It improves flexibility of RBCs and reduces viscosity of the blood. This improves microcirculation in ischemic areas. It is clinically used to establish circulation of affected areas. To some extent it also reduces platelet aggregation. It is indicated in nonhemorrhegic stroke, cerebrovascular disorders with transient ischemic attacks, intermittent claudication and leg ulcers. Dose 400 mg BD or TDS oral or IV

Pentoxyphylline improves flexibility of RBCs and reduces viscosity of the blood.

ISCHEMIC HEART DISEASES (IHD)

These disorders are characterized by myocardial impairment due to imbalance between myocardial oxygen demand and coronary blood supply. IHD are presented as angina pectoris, myocardial infarction (MI), cardiomyopathy or cardiac arrest .

In following situations heart demands more oxygen

1) Increased peripheral resistance: (increased afterload). Heart has to pump blood against more pressure. Ex. Hypertension.
2) Increased heart rate and increased force of contraction of heart: These situations increase work of heart.
3) Increased venous return (increased preload): heart has to pump more amount of the blood.

IHDs are characterized by imbalance between myocardial oxygen demand and coronary blood supply. They are presented as Angina pectoris, MI, cardiac arrest, etc.

In following situations heart gets less oxygen

1) Anemia: less oxygen content in blood
2) Tachycardia: Increased heart rate reduces diastolic period. Short diastolic period does not allow complete filling of blood and subsequently the blood flow to coronary vessels is reduced.
3) Arterial disorders

ANGINA PECTORIS

It is ischemic heart disorder that is characterized by substernal pain with heaviness. The pain radiates to arm, back and occipital region. The reason for angina, similar to IHD, is the increased demand of oxygen by heart or reduced supply of oxygen to myocardium.

Angina pectoris is of three types

1) Stable angina

This type of angina is precipitated by physical effort, emotional stress or sexual intercourse and is relieved by rest (also called classical angina).

Angina pectoris is of three types: stable, unstable and varient.

2) Unstable angina

This type of angina is usually associated with MI. It can be present at rest and symptoms are more severe and more frequent than classical angina.

3) Prinzmetal or variant angina

This type of angina is due to spasm of coronary arteries. The spasm usually is due to increased adrenergic activity or platelet aggregation. It is present commonly at night or early morning and at rest.

Management of angina

Objectives of management

1) To treat attack of angina
2) To reduce oxygen demand of heart (by reducing preload or afterload)
3) To prevent complications like MI.
4) To improve exercise tolerance.

Nonpharmacological measures

1) Explaining the patient about nature of the disease and altering life style.
2) Avoiding smoking, alcohol, stress.
3) Cardioprotective diet and exercises.

Figure 4.13 Drugs used in management of angina

Drugs used in management of angina

- Nitrates
  - Nitroglycerine
  - Isosorbide mononitrate
  - Isosorbide dinitrate
- Calcium channel blockers
  - Nifedipine
- β blockers
  - Metoprolol
  - Atenolol
- Miscellaneous
  - Dipyridamole
  - Aspirin
  - Nicorandil
  - Trimetazidine

Nitrates: (Refer Page 144).

Nitrates dilate veins, reduce venous return and filling of heart. Thus by reducing preload, they reduce oxygen demand. Additionally, they dilate coronary vessels and improve cardiac blood flow and also relieve spasm. Some arterial dilatation is also provided by nitrates. They are drugs of choice in treatment and prophylaxis of all types of angina.

Nitrates mainly act on veins, Beta-blockers on heart and CCBs on arteries.

(Dose: 0.3-0.6 mg sublingual nitrate for immediate relief, 2.5-15 mg oral nitroglycerine for maintenance). Ointments or patches also can be used to avoid tolerance. Long acting nitrates are avoided. Nitrates cause tachycardia by reflex sympathetic stimulation.

Nitrates are drugs of choice in angina of all types.

Calcium channel blockers: (Refer Page 141).

Calcium channel blockers dilate arteries and reduce peripheral resistance. Thus by reducing afterload they reduce oxygen demand of heart. Additionally some of them reduce contractability of heart. By dilating coronary arteries, CCBs improve cardiac blood supply. They are used along with nitrates or with β blockers. CCBs cause tachycardia and palpitations by reflex sympathetic stimulation. Dose: sublingual or oral nifedipine 10-30 mg, Amlodipine 2.5-10 mg

β blockers: β blockers, by blocking β_1 receptors on heart, reduce rate and contractability of heart and reduce work load and oxygen demand of heart. But they can increase coronary spasm in variant angina. Cardioselective agents usually are preferred in angina

Metoprolol: 50-100 mg OD or BD   Atenolol: 50-100 mg OD or BD

They are used in combination with nitrates in prophylaxis of stable angina.

Dipyridamole: (Refer page 168)

Adenosine is a regulator of coronary blood flow. Dipyridamole prevents its degradation and improves coronary blood flow. (25-100 mg TDS)

Aspirin: (Refer page 168). Aspirin, in low doses, prevents platelet aggregation and reduces the chances of clot formation and MI.

Nicorandil: It is a K channel opener and provides advantages like venodilatation (decreased preload), arterial dilatation (decreased afterload) and improvement in coronary blood flow.

Trimetazidine dihydrochloride: It increases uptake of lactate and pyruvic acid from ischemic area and reduces pain.

Rationale behind combinations

Nitrates, CCBs, and β blockers are used in combinations in management of angina (either only two or all three). The rationale for the combinations is:

1) Reflex tachycardia caused by nitrates or CCBs is compensated by β blockers.

2) Reduced coronary blood flow caused by β blockers is compensated by nitrates or CCBs.

3) Verapamil or diltiazem like CCBs are never combined with β blockers as all of them depress heart.

Management line in stable angina

Acute attack of angina

↓

Sublingual nitroglycerine or sublingual nifedipine

↓

Stop all activities immediately -bed rest

↓

If no relief from symptoms

↓

Repeat dose. If signs of overdose are seen spit out the sublingual tablet or swallow

↓

For Maintenance

Nonpharmacological measures like diet, moderate exercise, alcohol and smoking restriction is essential. For long-term prophylaxis: long acting nitrates can be used but they cause tolerance so they are used intermittently. CCBs or β blockers or nitrates are used as monotherapy or in combination of 2 or 3, depending on the control of attacks.

Combinations of nitrates, CCBs, and β blockers take care of limitations of each others.

Sublingual nitroglycerine or nifedipine is used prophylacticaly before exercise.

Unstable angina

Unstable angina is a medical emergency and the major objective of treatment is to prevent thrombosis and MI

Unstable angina is a medical emergency

Hospitalization-bed rest

↓

Sedation- with pethidine

↓

Sublingual or IV nitroglycerine till relief.

↓

Aspirin and/or heparin is administered to prevent thrombus formation. Additionally, CCBs or β blockers can also be given

Prinzmetal angina

The major objective is to relieve the spasm and immediate treatment is crucial. Sublingual nitroglycerine or nifedipine.

↓

If no relief - repeat the same

↓

Maintenance on sustained release nifedipine

Silent ischemia: It is the objective conformation of ischemia without the signs and symptoms. This is usually diagnosed on investigations.

MANAGEMENT OF CARDIAC FAILURE

(HEART FAILURE)

It is the condition in which heart cannot pump sufficient amount of the blood i.e. the amount required by all organs in the body. In other words it is abnormality of myocardial function that is responsible for failure of heart to pump blood in the amount that is sufficient for body requirement. Forward failure is lack of pumping of sufficient amount of blood while backward failure is mainly due to dumping of blood and increased back pressure .Inadequate perfusion of organs, systemic edema, pulmonary edema due to congestion are major problems associated with CCF. Acute left ventricular failure is sudden inability of heart to maintain cardiac output and BP. It results in sudden reflex arterial and venous constriction. Back pressure on pulmonary vein produces pulmonary edema and there is breathlessness especially orthopnea.

Cardiac failure is inability of heart to pump sufficient amount of blood.

Objectives of management

1) Reducing morbidity and mortality
2) Reducing afterload
3) Reducing preload and edema
4) Improving contractions of heart
5) Treatment of associated conditions
6) Prevention of complications

Nonpharmacological management

Rest, salt restricted diet, moderate fluid restriction, weight control are some of the crucial issues in nonpharmacological management. Drugs used in management of cardiac failure are as follows:

Figure 4.14 Drugs used in management of cardiac failure

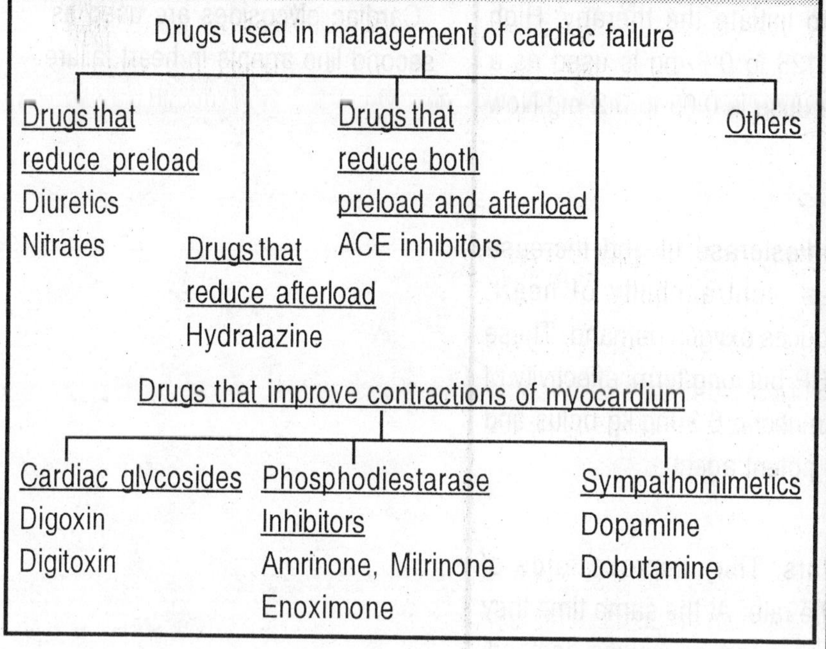

Diuretics: (Refer page 150). Diuretics, by increasing diuresis, promote loss of water and electrolytes and reduce preload by reducing venous return. They reduce pulmonary and systemic edema. Thiazides or loop diuretics are used as first line agents in the management of cardiac failure. Potassium sparing diuretics are coupled with them to compensate potassium loss.

Frusemide	-	40-120 mg oral (in severe failure)
Hydrochlorthiazide	-	25-200 mg (in mild failure)
Spironolactone	-	50-200 mg oral
Amiloride	-	5-20 mg

Diuretics achieve reduction in venous return. Diuretics reduce pulmonary and systemic edema.

Nitrates: (Refer page 144).

Nitrates dilate veins and reduce venous return and ventricular filling pressure. They prevent ventricular stretching. This reduces oxygen demand of heart. Nitroglycerine 2.5 to 20 mg sustained release tablets or isosorbide dinitrate (5-40 mg) or isosorbide mononitrate (10-20 mg).

Nitrates reduce preload.

ACE inhibitors: (Refer page 138). These are the most effective vasodilators. They act on arteries and veins and reduce preload and afterload, almost without increase in reflex sympathetic activity. Other vasodilators (due to reflex sympathetic activation) increase heart rate, raise PR and increase oxygen demand of heart.

Dose: Enalapril: 2.5-20 mg OD-BD, lisinopril 5-40 mg OD

Hydralazine: Hydralazine, by generating NO, dilates arteries and reduces afterload. This reduces work load of heart. But reflex sympathetic activation with hydralazine increases work load on heart.

Dose: 10-100 mg oral or 5-10 mg IM or IV.

ACE inhibitors reduce preload and afterload without reflex sympathetic stimulation.

Cardiac glycosides: (Refer page 147).

Cardiac glycosides improve contractibility of heart, improve ejection fraction and cardiac output. This action is achieved without increase in heart rate. In a way cardiac function is improved without increase in oxygen demand of heart. Cardiac glycosides have narrow therapeutic range. Digoxin is the preferred agent to initiate the therapy. High loading dose is required, then usually 0.125 to 0.5 mg is used as a maintenance dose. Digitoxin maintenance dose is 0.05 to 0.2 mg Now they are not used as first line therapy.

Cardiac glycosides are used as second line agents in heart failure.

Phosphodiesterase III inhibitors

These agents inhibit enzyme phosphodiesterase III and increase accumulation of cAMP. This improves contractibility of heart. Vasodilatation caused by these agents reduces oxygen demand. These agents have less effect on heart rate and BP, but long-term effectivity of these agents is not established. Dose: Amrinone 0.5 mg/kg bolus and then 5-10 μg/kg/min. Milrinone is a more potent agent.

Sympathomimetic agents

These agents act on D and β receptors. They improve force of contraction of heart but do not increase the rate. At the same time they reduce peripheral resistance. All these factors reduce oxygen demand. Additionally, these drugs improve renal blood flow and protect kidneys.

Dopamine IV 2.5-50 μg/kg/min

Dobutamine IV 2.5 - 10 μg/kg/min

Dopamine and dobutamine improve contractile function of heart, at the same time maintain renal blood flow.

Drugs like hydralazine (arterial vasodilators), prazosin (α_1 blocker) and some β blockers are also used rarely in cardiac failure.

Management line

CCF

↓

Start with nonpharmacological management

↓

If not controlled, thiazide diuretics + K sparing diuretics + ACE inhibitors (or) Loop diuretics + spironolactone

↓

If not controlled

↓

Proper combination of diuretics + ACE inhibitors + cardiac glycosides.

Nitrates, hydralazine or prazosin can be used at any stage (but not as first line) depending on doctor and patient.

Amrinone, milrinone and sympathomimetics are used for short term reliefs.

Management of acute left ventricular failure:

Treatment of pulmonary edema is crucial in LVF. Steps in management:

Semi upright posture and oxygen

Controlling venous return and reduction in fluid is a primary goal. It is achieved by

i) applying tourniquets

ii) loop diuretics - (reduce fluid overload).

iii) Nitrates (produce vasodilatation).

iv) Opioid analgesics (relieve distress and breathlessness).

v) Aminophylline (relieves bronchospasm).

In acute LVF, treatment of pulmonary edema is crucial.

MANAGEMENT OF HYPERTENSION

Hypertension is persistent high arterial blood pressure.

Stages of hypertension		
	Systolic	**Diastolic**
Normal	<130	<85
High normal	130-139	85-89
Stage 1 (mild)	140-159	90-99
Stage 2 (moderate)	160-179	100-109
Stage 3 (severe)	180-209	110-119
Stage 4 (very severe)	>210	>120
Isolated systolic	>160	-

Objectives of management

1) Keeping BP under control for 24 hours

2) Preventing complications like MI, retinopathy, stroke, coronary heart diseases, renal failure.

4) Reduction in morbidity and mortality

5) Investigating and treating cause

Nonpharmacological management

Nonpharmacological measures are essential in management of hypertension.

1) Restrict smoking and oral tobacco to prevent peripheral vascular disorders.

2) Regular physical exercise to reduce sympathetic overactivity and to reduce weight.

3) Biofeedback meditation: to reduce stress.

4) Diet to control weight and lipids.

Drugs used in management of HT

Various drugs are available for pharmacological management of HT. They reduce blood pressure by different mechanisms. The choice of drugs depends on the individual patient.

Refer figure 4.15 on page 176.

Figure 4.15 Drugs available for pharmacological management of HT

Drugs used in management of HT

- ACE Inhibitors: Captopril, Lisinopril, Enalapril
- Calcium channel blockers: Nifedipine, Amlodipine
- Angiotensin antagonist: Losartan
- Centrally acting agents: Clonidine, α methyl dopa
- β blockers: Atenolol, Metoprolol, Propranolol
- Diuretics: Hydrochlorthiazides, Chlorthiazide, Indapamide
- Vasodilators: Hydralazine, Nitroprusside, Diazoxide
- α Blockers: Prazosin, Terazosin

Mechanisms by which these drugs provide benefits in hypertension:

ACE inhibitors: (Refer page 138). These agents act by reducing formation of angiotensin. They

a) Reduce peripheral resistance by vasodilatation.

b) Potentiate bradykinin mediated vasodilatation.

c) Reduce cardiac hypertrophy.

d) Inhibit action of aldosterone and reduce fluid and Na retention. They are preferably used in HT associated with angina and MI, diabetic nephropathy, hyperlipidemias, high renin activity and young age. They are usually avoided in pregnancy and renal artery stenosis. Cough is a major side effect. Dose: lisinopril 5-40 mg OD, Enalapril 2.5-20 mg OD.

ACE inhibitors are preferred in HT with angina, MI, diabetic nephropathy, high renin activity and left ventricular hypertrophy.

β blockers: (Refer Page 99).

These agents block β receptors and reduce force of contraction of heart and cardiac output. Additionally they have the action that reduces peripheral resistance. They also have antirenin activity. Cardioselective agents are with intrinsic sympathetic activity usually preferred. β blockers are preferred in younger age group and in HT associated with anxiety, tachycardia, angina or in post MI hypertension. They are avoided in asthma, heart block, hyperlipidemias and diabetes. These agents are very cheap and can be given in pregnancy. Atenolol 50-100 mg OD, Metoprolol 50-100 mg BD.

Beta blockers are preferred in HT with anxiety and tachycardia.

Diuretics: (Refer page 150).

Diuretics reduce fluid overload and reduce cardiac output. Additionally, these agents reduce peripheral resistance and reduce sensitivity of blood vessel to Na and reduce BP .Diuretics are preferred in elderly population, HT with edema, in low renin activity and in renal disorders with Na retention. They are usually avoided in diabetes, hyperlipidemias and in pregnancy.

Chlorthiazide	-	125-250 mg/day
Indapamide	-	2.5-5 mg/day

Diuretics are preferred in HT with obesity, low renin activity and Na retention.

Calcium channel blockers: (Refer page 141).

These drugs block calcium channels in the cells. They reduce entry of calcium in cells and cause relaxation of blood vessels. As their major action is on arteries, they reduce peripheral resistance and blood pressure. CCBs are preferred in elderly population and in HT associated with asthma, COPD (chronic obstructive pulmonary disorder) and peripheral vascular disorders. They are usually avoided in ventricular hypertrophy. Dose: Amlodipine 2.5-10 mg OD, nifedipine 30-120 mg/day.

Above mentioned four classes of drugs are used as first line agents in the management of HT. Some other drugs that can be used along with it are:

CCBs are preferred in HT associated with COPD and peripheral vascular disorders.

Angiotensin antagonists: (Refer page 141). These drugs block angiotensin receptor and produce response like ACE inhibitors. Recently, they are being used as first line agents. Ex. Losartan 50 mg OD or BD.

Centrally acting agents : (Refer Page 179).

These agents act on α receptors in CNS and reduce overall sympathetic tone and reduce blood pressure.

Clonidine: 100 mcg OD or BD max 300 mcg oral or IM

α methyldopa: 250-500 mg BD-QID oral

Clonidine and alpha methyldopa act predominantly in CNS and reduce blood pressure.

α blockers block α receptors, produce vasodilatation and subsequent reduction in PR and BP. Dose: Prazosin 1-5 mg BD.

Hydralazine: It, by dilating arteries, reduces PR and BP. Dose: 25-50 mg BD-TDS.

Nitroprusside: It has transient vasodilator action. Dose: 0.25 μg/kg/min IV.

Rationale for combination of antihypertensive agents

1) Combinations, as far as possible ,should be avoided and patients are to be maintained on monotherapy. This improves compliance.

2) Loop diuretics or thiazides cause loss of K. So potassium sparing diuretics are combined with these agents.

3) Vasodilators like CCBs or nitrates or α blockers cause reflex tachycardia, which can be compensated by β blockers.

4) Sympatholytic agents (centrally and peripherally acting) cause fluid retention. Addition of diuretics reduce retention and so the tolerance.

5) Synergistic action is observed between ACE inhibitors and diuretics

Management line in hypertension

Nonpharmacological management is a crucial issue in hypertension. A large number of drugs are available for treatment of hypertension and choice depends on individual patient. This is termed as individualized therapy. Drug of choice depends upon various factors like severity, age of patient, associated conditions and cost of treatment. Following are commonly used guidelines but not rigid criteria to decide the choice of drug.

Figure 4.16 Stages and treatment of HT

Patient of HT

Stage 1
↓
Nonpharmacological management
↓
No response for 3-6 month
↓
Pharmacological treatment (monotherapy)

Stage 2
↓
Nonpharmacological management
↓
Less waiting period (15 days to 1 month)
↓
Pharmacological treatment (monotherapy)

Stage 3
Nonphamarcological management
+
Monotherapy

Stage 4
Nonpharmacological management
+
Usually combination therapy.

Figure 4.17 Age and HT

Age

- Young patients: β blockers/ACE inhibitors
- Elderly: Diuretics/CCBs

Figure 4.18 Severity and HT

Severity

Mild
Monotherapy with
Diuretics or
CCBs or
ACE inhibitors or
β blockers or
Angiotensin antagonist

Moderate
First line agents in higher doses or different drugs or combinations

Severe
Using high doses or high dose combinations or adding second line agents

Emergency
(see below)

Treatment of hypertensive emergency

Hypertensive emergency is not only related to severity. It is the rise in BP that can cause encephalopathy, aneurism, eclampsia or left ventricular failure. It demands immediate reduction in BP. (within 1 minute to 4 hours, depending on condition).

Drugs used are

Nitroprusside	0.25 μg/kg/min IV
Diazoxide	50-150 mg IV over 5 minutes
Labetolol	20-80 mg IV over 3 - 6 hrs
Clonidine	100-300 μg/kg IV

In less urgent situations IV hydralazine or sublingual nitroglycerine can be used.

Hypertensive emergencies demand immediate reduction in hypertension.

Conditions associated with HT also govern drug of choice in HT

Conditions associated with HT also govern drug of choice in HT

Figure 4.19 Associated conditions and HT

Associated condition	Drug of choice
Anxiety and tachycardia	β blockers
Obesity	Diuretics
Diabetes with nephropathy	ACE inhibitors
Angina or MI	ACE inhibitors or β blockers
Asthma or COPD	CCBs
Hyperlipidemia	ACE inhibitors
LVF or ventricular hypertrophy	ACE inhibitors
Peripheral vascular disorders	CCBs
High renin HT	ACE inhibitors
Low renin HT	Diuretics
Renal disorders with Na retention	Diuretics

When cost is a concern, β blockers and diuretics are cheaper alternatives.

When HT is adequately controlled, investigations to find out and treat the cause are essential.

CENTRALLY ACTING ANTIHYPERTENSIVE AGENTS (CENTRAL SYMPATHOLYTICS)

These drugs reduce BP by their action in CNS. Ex. Clonidine and α methyldopa.

Clonidine

Mechanism of action:

1) Clonidine stimulates postsynaptic α_2 receptors in CNS and reduce overall sympathetic tone of the body.

2) It also stimulates presynaptic α_2 receptors in peripheral nerve endings and reduce release of noradrenaline and reduce PR. (Refer page 185).

3) It is proposed to act on specific imidazoline receptors which reduce sympathetic tone.

4) Clonidine has some analgesic action.

Indications

1) Moderate hypertension (not as a first line drug)
2) Hypertensive emergency,
3) As preanesthetic (to reduce dose of anesthetic agent) and post-op (to reduce pain)
4) Opioid withdrawal: In individuals with opioid addiction, opioid withdrawal is supported by clonidine treatment.

α Methyldopa

Mechanism of action

Mechanism of action of this drug is controversial. This agent is analogue of dopa (dopamine precursor). In CNS, it gets converted into α methyl NA.

α Methyl dopa
↓
α methyl NA
↓
Stimulation of α_2 receptors in CNS
↓
Decreased sympathetic tone
↓
Reduced PR and BP

α methyl dopa reduces overall sympathetic tone

Postural hypotension is not a problem with this drug.

Indication: Mild to moderate hypertension (It is not used in isolation but is used in combination with diuretics).

Side effects: Sedation, reduced mental activity, hypersensitivity.

Dose: 250 - 500 mg BD to QID

MANAGEMENT OF MYOCARDIAL INFARCTION

Myocardial infarction (MI)

It is the ischemic necrosis of myocardium due to coronary occlusion.

Objectives of management

1) Pain relief
2) Breaking down the clot in the coronary vessel
3) Prevention of further damage
4) Identifying and treating complications like arrhythmia, hypotension, shock.
5) Prevention of future attacks.

Management line

Line of management varies according to the hemodynamic and cardiovascular status of the patient. Certain standard guidelines are followed:

1) Morphine 5-10 mg IV or SC
(it reduces pain and anxiety. Not only it provides symptomatic relief but

also reduces overall sympathetic tone of the body

2) Oxygenation: To fulfil oxygen demand easily.

3) Streptokinase (1500000 units over one hour) or alteplase (10 mg bolus, 50 mg over 1 hr and 40 mg over next 2 hours) is administered within 6 hours to break the thrombus that is already formed. This can prevent possible damage due to that clot. Reestablishment of circulation is also achieved by these drug.

4) Aspirin 50-150 mg is administered to prevent platelet aggregation and reformation of clot

5) Oral anticoagulants can be used for long term prophylaxis.

Associated medications

Low molecular weight dextran: to increase plasma volume. Sodium bicarbonate: to prevent acidosis

Vasodilators (IV nitroglycerine): to reduce work load of heart

Diuretics (frusemide): to reduce fluid overload.

Antiarrhythmics: use of these agents depends on the situation.

LIPID LOWERING AGENTS

Excess lipids in body collect in blood vessels as atheroma. Blood vessels become narrow and loose elasticity. It reduces oxygenation of the area supplied by that vessel. Lipid lowering agents reduce harmful lipids and lipoproteins in the body. By lowering lipid levels, these agents reduce incidence of atherosclerotic disorders of coronary and cerebral vessels.

Atherosclerotic disorders are associated with high cholesterol and triglyceride levels.

Physiological considerations

Lipid metabolism is complex process and can't be discussed in details here. But essential facts that are required to understand pharmacology of lipid lowering agents are illustrated here and at appropriate places in this section.

Plasma lipids are present in four forms

i) Cholesterol (CH)

ii) Triglycerides (TG)

iii) Phospholipids (PL)

iv) Free fatty acids (FFA)

HDL are protective lipoproteins, all others are harmful.

All these lipids, in plasma, combine with apolipoproteins to form lipoproteins. Lipoproteins, depending on their density, are classified as HDL, LDL, IDL, VLDL and chylomicrons.

HDL: High density lipoproteins: These lipoproteins predominantly contain PL and proteins and are responsible for transport of cholesterol from tissues to liver. (CH or TG when is transported away from the tissues into liver the chances of vascular abnormalities are reduced). So these are actually protective lipoproteins.

LDL: Low density lipoproteins: LDL mainly contain CH and are involved in transporting cholesterol into tissues and liver.

IDL: Intermediate density lipoproteins: IDL mainly contains CH and some TG. IDL is the source of LDL.

VLDL: Very low density lipoproteins: VLDL mainly contain TG and are responsible for transport of TG from liver (where TG are synthesized) to various tissues.

Chylomicrons: Chylomicrons are lipoproteins with minium density. These are involved in transport of dietary triglycerides to tissues.

Hyperlipidemia is basically classified as

i) Primary: It is of genetic origin

ii) Secondary: associated with alcoholism, diabetes mellitus, hypothyroidism, chronic liver diseases, nephrotic syndrome, drug induced, etc.

Hyperlipidemias of primary type are further divided in following manners.

Type IIb and type IV are common hyperlipidemic disorders.

Type I : This is a rare type of disorders. It is characterized by deficiency of enzyme lipoprotein lipase. This enzyme is responsible for utilization of TG and chylomicrons. Its deficiency results in elevated levels of CH, TG and chylomicron. This lipoproteinemia is not associated with atherosclerotic disorder.

Type IIa : Comparatively common: it is characterized by less number of LDL receptors in the liver. It results in reduced uptake of LDL from blood. It results in **V LDL** and CH. It is associated with heart diseases.

Type IIb : This is common and is characterized by increased LDL, VLDL, cholesterol and TG. Risk of IHD is very high with this type of disorder.

Type III : This is rare and is due to inherent abnormal lipoprotein (broad beta lipoprotein). It results in increased CH, TG and IDL. It is associated with heart diseases and peripheral vascular disorders

Except type I, all types are associated with atherosclerotic disorders.

Type IV : It is common and is characterized by high TG and VLDL and associated with heart diseases.

Type V : It is uncommon and is characterized by high TG, CH, VLDL and chylomicron. It is associated with high chances of heart diseases.

Table 4.12 Type of hyperlipidemias and predominant elevations

Type	Predominant elevations
I	TG, Chylomicrons
II_a	CH, LDL
II_b	TG, CH, LDL, VLDL
III	TG, CH, IDL, LDL.
IV	TG, VLDL
V	TG, CH, VLDL, Chylomicrons

Except for the first, almost all are associated with heart diseases.

Management of hyperlipidemias

Objectives of management

i) Keeping levels of lipids and lipoproteins within recommended limits

CH	<	200 mg/dl
TG	<	150 mg/dl
LDL	<	130 mg/dl
HDL	>	40 mg/dl

ii) Close watch over coronary heart disorders

iii) Searching and treating associated disorders including pancreatitis.

Nonpharmacological management is crucial in hyperlipidemic disorders.

Nonpharmacological management

It is very crucial in hyperlipidemias and many patients can be stabilized with it.

i) Reduction in smoking and alcohol

ii) Weight control

iii) Regular exercise

iv) Diet: Only 30% of total calories should come from fats. Daily diet must contain around 30 gm of fibres. Sugar consumption is reduced if there is increase in triglycerides (as there is a risk of pancreatitis).

Figure 4.20 Drugs used in management of hyperlipidemias

Drugs used in management of hyperlipidemias

- Resins
  - Cholestyramine
  - Colestipol
- HMGCoA reductase inhibitors
  - Lovastatin
  - Simvastatin
  - Pravastatin
  - Fluvastatin
- Fibric acid derivatives
  - Gemfibrozil
  - Clofibrate
  - Fenofibrate
- Nicotinic acid derivatives
  - Nicotinic acid
  - Acipimox
- Miscellaneous
  - Probucol
  - Omega-3- fatty acid
  - Marine triglycerides

All agents reduce cholesterol and LDL
All agents except resins reduce VLDL
All agents increase HDL

All agents reduce cholesterol and LDL
All agents except resins reduce VLDL
All agents increase HDL

Drug therapy once initiated, is life long.

Resins

These are bile acid binding agents that reduce mainly cholesterol and LDL, Ex. Cholestyramine and colestipol

Mechanism of action

Cholesterol is formed in liver. A part of that cholesterol is secreted along with bile into intestines and reabsorbed into blood. Resins, after oral administration bind to bile acids in intestines and prevent reabsorption of cholesterol. Due to lack of absorption of bile, there is compensatory increase in bile synthesis and more cholesterol from plasma is utilized.

Oil depletion of cholesterol in liver demands more cholesterol in liver. To get more CH in liver, LDL receptors upregulation takes place and cholesterol from plasma is brought to liver.

Resins reduce cholesterol and LDL and are used when triglyceride levels are normal.

Net effects: Reduction in CH and LDL. Increase in TG. No change in VLDL.

These agents are available as powders and taken once or twice a day with meals.

Indications: First line agents for hypercholesterolemia. (IIa/IIb/V)

Limitations

i) These agents are not used when TG levels are increased (as resins can increase TG)

ii) Unpalatability of these agents reduce compliance: to avoid this, they are used with fruit juice or are mixed with food.

iii) GI complaints like constipation, bloating, indigestion are responsible for reduced compliance.

iv) Resins are not effective in biliary obstruction.

Individual agents: Cholestyramine 4-24 gm/day. Colestipol 5-30 gm/day. Both drugs are taken with meals in 1-2 doses.

HMGCoA reductase inhibitors

HMGCoA is 3-hydroxy methyl glutaryl coenzyme A.

These agents are most widely used agents in hyperlipidemias. Ex. Statins: Lovastatin, simvastatin, fluvastatin, atrovastatin.

Mechanism of action

1) Cholesterol is synthesized in liver from acetyl CoA. The synthesis involves number of reactions, out of which conversion of HMGCoA into mevalonates is a rate limiting step. HMGCoA reductase is the enzyme that stimulates this step. HMGCoA reductase inhibitors inhibit enzyme HMGCoA reductase and reduce synthesis of cholesterol in liver.

2) Reduction in CH in liver demands more cholesterol in liver for which LDL receptors in the liver are up-regulated and LDL from plasma comes to liver.

HMGCoA reductase inhibitors are commonly used when cholesterol levels are increased.

Net effect: These agents produce marked reduction in CH, LDL, VLDL. Some reduction in TG and increase in HDL.

Indications

These agents are used when there is predominant rise in cholesterol and are preferred in types: IIa, IIb and V.

Adverse effects: These drugs are comparatively safe but transient alterations in LFTs, prolongation of prothrombin time, reversible muscle pain, GI disturbances, dizziness, vision problem are some adverse effects with statins.

Table 4.13 HMGCoA reductase inhibitors

Individual agents and dose	Features
Lovastastin 10-80 mg/day	Twice a day with meals
Pravastatin 5-40 mg/day	Once a day with evening meals
Simvastatin 5-40 mg/day	More potent. Once a day with evening meals
Atrovastatin Fluvastatin 20-80 mg/day	More potent. Reduces TG also

Fibrates

These are fibric acid derivatives and have wide spectrum of hypolipidemic activities. Ex. Gemfibrozil, clofibrate, bezafibrate, fenofibrate.

Mechanism of action

i) TG are synthesized in liver with the help of FFA. Fibrates inhibit release of FFA from adipose tissue and reduce formation of hepatic TG and that of VLDL.

ii) Lipoprotein lipase is the enzyme that hydrolyses TG in VLDL into FFA and glycerol. Fibrates stimulates activity of this enzyme and convert TG into FFA and glycerol. The net effects is reduction in TG and VLDL.

Fibrates predominantly reduce triglyceride levels.

4) Fibrates stimulate binding of peripheral LDL to LDL receptors in liver and reduce peripheral LDL and CH.

5) These agents also reduce HMGCoA and inhibit synthesis of CH.

6) These agents also reduce fibrinogen levels and promote fibrinolysis

Net effect: Predominant reduction in TG and VLDL. Some reduction in CH and LDL. Increase in HDL

These agent are used when CH or TG are increased individually or together. Fibrates are effective in II, IV, V hyperlipidemias as first line agents and as adjuvants in II_b, III

These agent are used when CH or TG are increased individually or together.

Adverse effects: Nausea, abdominal discomfort, loss of libido, muscle weakness. They are contraindicated in hepatic and renal impairments.

Table 4.14 Fibrates

Individual agents and dose	Features
Gemfibrozil 900-1200 mg before food	Found to reduce incidence of nonfatal MI
Bezafibrate 200 mg TDS	It additionally sensitizes action of insulin and so preferred in diabetes mellitus.
Clofibrate 1.5-2 gm/day	Increased risk of gallstone formation

Fibrates are usually not combined with statins because both the agents cause muscle pain.

Nicotinic acid derivatives (Niacin)

Niacin is Vit B, but in pharmacological doses it acts as a hypolipidemic agent.

Mechanism of action

Similar to fibrates, it inhibits release of FFAs from adipose tissues and reduces its availability for synthesis of TG in liver.

Net effects: Predominant reduction in TG, some reduction in CH, LDL and VLDL, increase in HDL.

Nicotinic acid predominantly reduces TG

Indications: These agents are used when TG are elevated or when both TG and CH are elevated (Type II/IV/V)

Adverse Effects: More common. Vasodilatation, flushing, GI discomfort pruritus, glucose intolerance, headache, altered LFTs, etc.

Table 4.15 Nicotinic acid derivatives

Individual agents and dose	Features
Niacin 100 mg TDS-up to 6 gm	Side effects limit its use
Acipimox 1200 mg in divided doses with meals	Longer acting and less side effects

Side effects limit use of niacin

Miscellaneous agents

Probucol: It is structurally different than other antihyperlipidemics. It is basically an antioxidant. It prevents oxidation of fatty acids in lipoproteins due to which ability of endothelial cells to take up LDL is reduced. (Dose: 500 mg BD with meals). It has got no effects on TG but it reduces LDL predominantly. In hyperlipidemias that are resistant and with high VLDL level, probucol is used as an adjuvant. Gastrointestinal abnormalities like diarrhea, flatulence and ventricular arrhythmias are side effects, which limit the use of drug in cardiac patients.

Omega 3 fatty acids: These agents improve peripheral clearance of VLDL and reduce synthesis of TG in liver. The combination available contains eicosapentaenoic acid (EPA). 180 mg and decosahepaenoic acid 120 mg. Dose: is 3-12 capsules per day.

Hormone replacement therapy: (Estrogen + Progesterone) is used in menopausal women. HRT reduces LDL levels but increases TG levels.

Line of management

Nonpharmacological management is very crucial. Drugs are not started unless nonpharmacological measures fail in moderate cases because drug treatment once started is required throughout the life. Drug therapy depends on affected lipids or lipoproteins.

I) Hypertriglyceridemia

'Fibrates' or Fibrates + low dose nicotinic acid or omega 3 fatty acids.

II) Hypercholesterolemia

Start with low doses of statins (HMGCoA reductase inhibitors): If not controlled add resins. Alternative to statins is fibrates, but are not as effective as statins..

III) Hypertriglyceridemia + Hypercholesterolemia

If CH rise predominant: Use statins

If TG rise predominant: Use fibrates

Nicotinic acid can be used in all conditions.

Probucol or omega 3 proteins are used as adjuvants in resistant cases.

Guidelines for using drugs

	CH	TG	VLDL	LDL	HDL
Resins	-2	+1	–	-2	+1
Statins	-3	-1	-3	-3	+1
Fibrates	-1	-3	-3	-1	+2
Nicotinic Acid	-1	-3	-1	-1	+1

(-) indicates reduction, (+) indicates rise, 1-4 indicate magnitude.

CARDIAC ARRHYTHMIAS

by Dr.SHASHANK SHROTRIYA

Chaos of the rhythmic beating of heart is called as arrhythmia. Like any other chaos, this is potentially morbid and sometimes fatal. However, ignorance about its management can be fatal. This is one such area where the physician must remember, "Let the drug be less dangerous than the abnormal rhythm." Most anti-dysrrhythmic drugs may have depressive action of myocardial activity and some times lead to arrhythmias themselves. This makes the selection of drug a delicate process.

Chaos of the rhythmic beating of heart is called as arrhythmia.

Physiological basis of arrhythmia

Every muscle in the heart contracts or relaxes, after an impulse is given.

Impulse is electrical current. This current depends upon the potential difference between charges. These charges are in the form of quantity of ions present across the cell membrane of individual cells. In normal resting stage, the inside of a cell is negatively charged. Stimulus leads to movement of positive ions across the membrane. This potential difference leads to generation of an impulse that is called as action potential. This action potential then spreads to the adjacent cell, which is called as conductivity. Ability of some part of the cardiac cells to generate an action potential without any stimulus is called as automaticity. The sinoatrial node (SA) is called as pacemaker of heart. The impulse from SA node travels from the atria to ventricles, in between them is atrioventricular (AV) node. The delay due to AV conduction gives the heart a logical contraction of the ventricles after the contraction of atrium. This is very important in maintaining a proper cardiac output. Purkinje fibres and bundle of His are present in ventricles. They are conducting systems. Now let us see the action potential of heart, the different phases and the movement of NA$^+$, K$^+$ & Ca$^+$ across a cell membrane.

Figure 4.21 Action potential

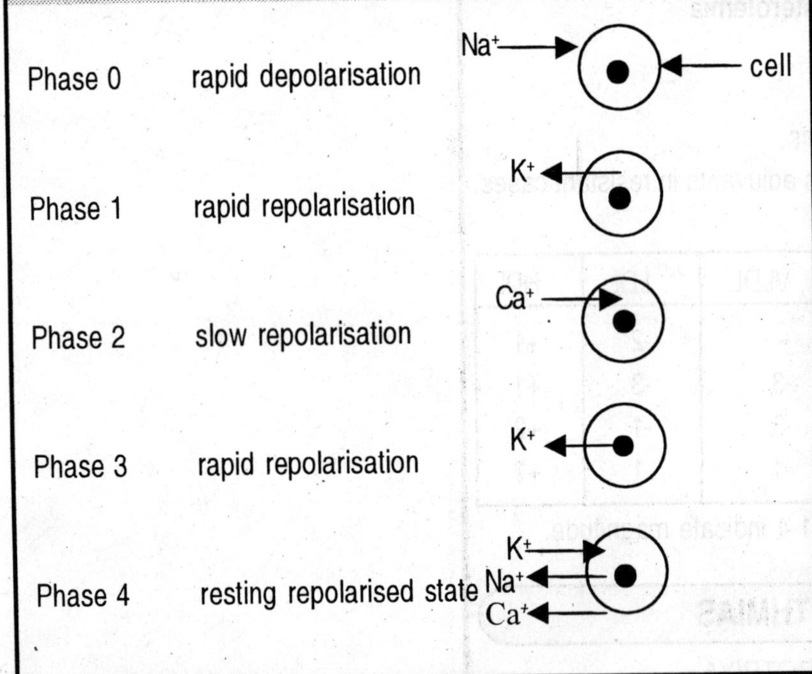

The above picture shows five different phases of action potential and four different classes of antiarrhythmic drugs.

Phase 0	rapid depolarization of cell
Phase 1	rapid repolarization
Phase 2	slow repolarization
Phase 3	rapid repolarization
Phase 4	resting repolarized state

Phase 0 is when an impulse causes opening of the Na$^+$ channels and there is influx of the Na$^+$ inside the cell. This will lead to create a positive charge across the cell membrane. This is called as depolarization.

Phase 1 is when there is a small but rapid efflux of the K^+ from the cell. This is the start of repolarization.

Phase 2 is when the repolarization becomes slow due to slow influx of Ca+ inside the cell.

Phase 3 is when there is complete repolarization of the cell membrane due to efflux of the K^+ from the cell. This is an active process and needs ATP. This is possible due to a Na^+K^+ pump.

Phase 4 is when the cell restores its original ionic position. The Na^+ ions come out of the cell and the K^+ ions go back in the cell. Ca^+ ions also come out of the cell and the cell becomes once again ready for the next action potential to generate.

Phase 1 & 2 are called as absolute refractory period where the cell cannot be further responded to any stimuli.

cell cannot be further responded to any stimuli in absolute refractory period

Phase 3 is called as relative refractory period when cell will once again depolarized in the wake of an unusually strong stimulus.

CLASSIFICATION OF DYSRRHYTHMIAS

A) Abnormal automaticity

When the pacemaker gets excited abnormally, this leads to abnormally high rate called as tachycardia, untimely contraction of atrium and ventricles called extra systoles or atrial flutter (where atrium beats up to 250 beats/min). This can be due to post-myocardial infarction injury.

B) Untimely depolarization

1) During phase 3 (i.e. relative refractory period), depolarization due to K^+ outflow obstruction will lead to bradycardia and abnormally long action potentials.

2) During phase 4, early depolarization, even before complete repolarization, has taken place. This may be due to Ca^+ overload, digitalis toxicity and will lead to premature ectopic beats that are seen on ECG.

C) Re-entry

Due to abnormal conduction, an impulse may recirculate and re-excite the original site, leading to abnormally high rate of action potential. There are two such patterns:

i) Circus movement type: when an impulse is obstructed unidirectional, it makes one-way transit across the obstacle, finds a new pathway and re-excites the original spot where it has generated. This leads to paroxysmal supra ventricular tachycardias (PSVT) and atrio-ventricular reciprocal tachycardias (WPW – Wolf Parkinson White Syndrome).

ii) Micro re-entry circuit: any block in the Purkinje Fibres in ventricle due to injury may lead to extremely slow conduction across that fibre. This will lead to reduced action potential duration and cause reexcitation of the proximal fibre. This will lead to ventricular extra systoles (extrabeats), ventricular tachycardia or ventricular fibrillation (i.e. when ventricles beats > 250 beats / min and can neither fill with blood nor can throw the blood forward).

D) Breakdown of an impulse

Asynchronous excitation of different atrial fibres lead to ineffective contraction of the atrium leading to atrial fibrillation. This may happen in over distended atrium in mitral stenosis.

E) Heart block

Slowing of conduction through the SA node and AV node due to ischemic injury leads to heart block. There are three degrees of heart block depending upon the worsening of the delay of conduction from atrium to ventricle.

CLASSIFICATION OF ANTIARRHYTHMIC DRUGS

Class 1: Na^+ channel blockers

A) Drugs that lengthen AP duration and refractory period.

B) Drugs shorten AP duration and refractory period.

C) Negligible effect on AP duration and refractory period.

Class 2: Catecholamine blockers (β receptor antagonist) Decrease sympathetic tone

Class 3: Widening of APD & ERP

Class 4: Ca^+ channel blockers

CLASS I

They inhibit the movement of Na^+ conduction in phase '0' and prolong the repolarization in phase 3. This will lead to:

a) Delayed depolarization

b) Prolonged action potential duration

c) Increase in the absolute refractory period.

d) Suppressed AV conduction and prolonged P-R, QRS & QT.

Quinidine

This is an alkaloid from chinchona bark, a dextro isomer of quinine.

Apart from the above-mentioned actions it has strong antivagal actions:

It prevents re-enterant arrhythmias by decreasing the automaticity.

Prolonging the refractive period of action potential, depolarization is delayed therefore useful in terminating atrial fibrillation, atrial flutter or PSVT (paroxysmal supra ventricular tachycardias).

By prolonging the phase 3, it prevents premature beats and extra systoles.

Quinidine depresses myocardial contraction especially in a damaged heart.

It causes hypotension due to direct action on blood vessels.

It decreases the contractility of skeletal muscles.

Pharmacokinetics: absorbed in the intestines, 90% metabolized in liver, peak action 1-2 hrs and remains for 6-8 hrs.

Dose: Given orally or slow IV, heart rate should be monitored. Available as quinidine sulphate 200 mg tab and quinidine gluconate 800 mg/10 ml injection.

Adverse effects:

1) Sudden death due to AV block, ventricular fibrillation or cardiac failures.

2) Cinchonism: ringing in ears, deafness, vertigo, headache, delirium, visual changes, mental derangements.

3) Idiosyncrasy and hypersensitivity.

4) Toxicity in chronic liver disease.

Interactions:

1) Can cause digitalis toxicity

2) Diuretics causing hypokalemia can cause quinidine toxicity.

3) Vasodilators can increase hypotension with quinidine

4) Synergistic cardiac depression with K^+ salts and β blockers.

Procainamide:

Amide derivative of procaine. It differs from quinidine in following way:

1) It is less potent.

2) It has less negative role on myocardial contraction. It causes less AV-block.

3) Poor antivagal action.

4) No effect on blood pressure because no α-blockade.

Pharmacokinetics: It's acetylated into N-acetyl-procainamide which blocks K^+ channels and has no effect on Na^+ channel. Therefore it increases the ERP. There are naturally slow or fast acetylators of this drug and action may differ in individual.

Dose: 500 mg - 1 gm bolus dose orally or IM followed by 250 mg to 500 mg every 2 hrly.

Adverse effect:

- Cardiotoxicity similar to quinidine
- GIT symptoms
- Hypersensitivity
- Can cause systemic lupus erythematosus (SLE) like disease on chronic use.

Disopyramide:

More antivagal than quinidine but no α blockade. Better tolerated therefore used as maintenance therapy after cardioversion of AF & AFL.

SUB CLASS 1B

They block Na^+ channels but poor action on K^+ channels. They do not suppress AV conduction, action potential duration.

Ex. Lignocaine, mexiletine, tocainide, phenytoin.

Lignocaine:

Most commonly used local anesthetic, popular antiarrhythmic drug used in ICUs.

It prolongs depolarization and thus decreases automaticity more in damaged tissue than in normal. It causes decreased action potential duration. It increases conduction more in ventricular tissue and not in atrium; therefore very useful in post myocardial infarction arrhythmias.

Pharmacokinetics: Lignocaine is absorbed orally but due to high first pass effect, it's inactivated therefore IV route is preferred. Action lasts only for 10-20 minutes; metabolism is dependant on hepatic blood flow. Therefore t½ is prolonged in chronic hepatic failure.

Dose: 50-100 mg IV bolus followed by 20-30 mg, available as Xylocard or Gesicard which has no preservative in it.

Adverse effects: Dose dependent neurological effects.

Used in ventricular tachycardias, ectopics during anesthesia, post myocardial infarction arrhythmias during cardiac surgery.

Mexiletine:

Chemically and pharmacologically similar to lignocaine. It is a local anesthetic with oral antiarrhythmic action. It has more adverse effects than lignocaine, can cause serious AV blocks, bradycardia and hypotension, has many neurological side effects.

Dose: 400-600 mg loading dose followed by 150-200 mg TDS. It is used in ventricular arrhythmias as alternative to lignocaine in resistant cases.

Phenytoin:

Antiepileptic drug with specific antiarrhythmic action in digitalis toxicity where it improves AV conduction slowed by digitalis.

SUBCLASS IC

More Na^+ channel blockade and less K^+ channel blockade. They delay phase '0', AV conduction and ERP, they have proarrythmic activities and can cause sudden death. They are not marketed in India and have severe GIT, neurological and visual disturbances.

Ex. Flecainide, Propafenone.

CLASS II

They are β receptor blockers and suppress adrenergically induced ectopic activity.

Propranolol:

It blocks β stimulation in heart. It decreases automaticity of SA node and ectopic foci when they are induced adrenergically and not otherwise. It causes prolongation of AV node refractory period, therefore prevents paradoxical ventricular tachycardia while treating atrial flutter or fibrillation. Depression of cardiac activity can cause hypotension.

Dose: 20-80 mg oral BD/TDS can be given IV.

Used more in emotionally and exercise induced tachyarrhythmias, in atrial fibrillation along with digitalis, in patients with secondary thyrotoxicosis or pheochromocytomas where adrenergic tone is high.

It can cause severe bradycardia.

Other β blockers that are used are sotalol and esmolol.

CLASS III

This has more action on phase III of action potential i.e. repolarization due to movement of K^+ out of the cell. Action potential duration is widened and ERP (effective refractory period) is increased. The tissue remains refractory even after repolarization and therefore reentrant arrhythmias are terminated.

Amiodarone:

It increases ERP, prolong APD more in ectopic automaticity than in SA node. It inhibits Ca^+ channels in myocardium and has noncompetitive β adrenergic blocking property.

Pharmacokinetics: Slow GIT absorption and delayed action, IV route is faster, duration of action is very long with (up to 3-8 weeks).

Dose: 400-600 mg/day for few weeks followed by 100-200 mg OD for maintenance therapy.

Adverse effects: GIT upsets, photosensitization, corneal microdeposits and liver damage can occur, however pulmonary alveolitis and fibrosis of lung are serious complication.

Use: Due to adverse effects, it's used for resistant ventricular tachyarrhythmias.

Bretylium:

It is an antihypertensive with erratic oral absorption and tolerance, now used intravenously to abolish ventricular fibrillation not responding to electrical defibrillation. **Dose:** 5-10 mg IV bolus over 16 minutes and repeated 6-8 hrly in 3-5 mg IV.

CLASS IV

They are primarily Ca^+ channel blockers.

Verapamil:

It blocks L type Ca^+ channels and delays their recovery.

- It decreases SA automaticity resulting into bradycardia.
- It causes vasodilatation
- Prolongs AV nodal ERP, slows AV nodal conduction and reentry at AV node is prevented.
- Negative inotropic action.

Diltiazem:

The actions are same as verapamil but are milder than it and there fore it's seldom used in the treatment of arrhythmias, except in PSVT.

Drugs for paroxysmal supraventricular tachycardia

Apart from Ca^+ channel blockers, propranolol, digoxin or adenosine are the preferred drug now.

Adenosine:

It activates K^+ channels and causes membrane hyperpolarization. SA node depression leads to bradycardia. AV node conduction is slowed down and in the atrium the AP duration is slowed down.

Comparison with the other drugs is:

- Efficacy is better than verapamil.
- No hemodynamic effects, no hypotension, can be used with beta-blockers where verapamil is contraindicated.
- Action lasts only for 10-15 seconds therefore no adverse effects.
- Effective in arrhythmias resistant to verapamil.
- It is expensive and unavailable
- Cannot be used in recurrences.

Other drugs used for AV Block:

Atropine:

Used for AV block due to digitalis toxicity.

Sympathomimetics (Adrenaline, Isoprenaline) are used for partial heart block.

CHOICE OF ANTIARRHYTHMIC TREATMENT

In spite of all the electrophysiological advances and research in the field of pharmacology, antiarrhythmic treatment still remains empirical. Treating arrhythmias gives us a wide range of choices and this can be very confusing. The current guideline for the treatment of arrhythmias is given below. (Refer table 4.16 on page 195)

Table 4.16 Management of arrhythmias		
Arrhythmia	**Acute treatment**	**Chronic therapy and Prophylaxis**
Sinus tachycardia	Propranolol	-----
Sinus bradycardia	Anticholinergics	-----
Premature atrial beats	Propranolol Quinidine	Quinidino Procainamide Disopyramide
Paroxysmal supraventricular tachycardia	Adenosine Verapamil Digoxin	Digoxin Verapamil Quinidine
Atrial flutter	Cardioversion Verapamil Digitalis	Quinidine Digitalis Amiodorone
Atrial fibrillation	Cardioversion Verapamil Quinidine	Qunidine Digitalis Amioderone
Ventricular extrasystole	Lignocaine Procainamide Mexilefine	Quinidine Mexiletine
Digitalis induced arrhythmia	Lignocaine Phenytoin Propranolol	----
Ventricular fibrillation	Defibrillation Lignocaine Bretylium	Bretylium Procainamide Amioderone
Complete heart block	Atropine Isoprenaline	Pace maker

DRUGS IN GASTROINTESTINAL SYSTEM

"THIS SECTION CONTAINS"

ACID PEPTIC DISORDERS

Physiological considerations of acid secretion

Parietal cells in stomach secrete hydrochloric acid (HCl). Gastric acid secretion is governed by various receptors. Stimulation of muscarinic, histaminic and gastrin receptor on parietal cells increases acid secretion while stimulation of prostaglandin receptors reduces acid secretion. (see figure).

Stimulation of M, H_2 and G receptors increases acid secretion while that of PG receptors reduces acid secretion.

Figure 5.1 Acid secretion

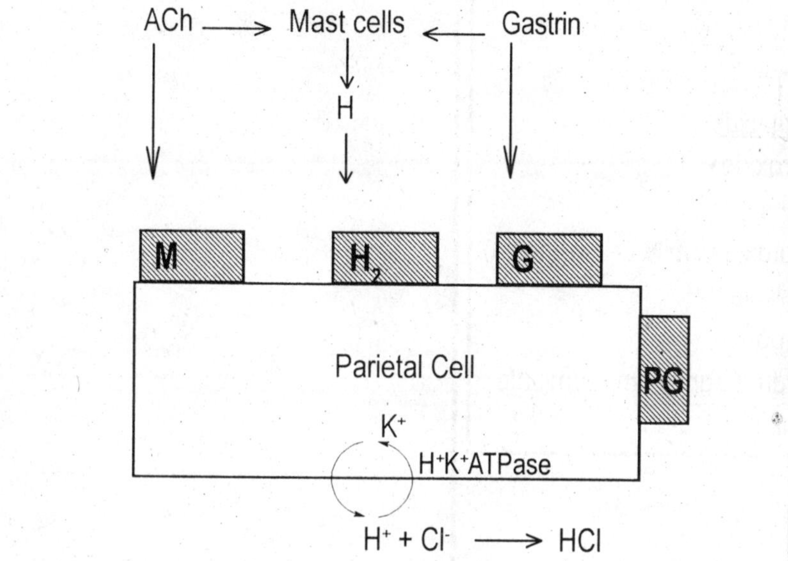

M	-	Muscarinic receptors.
H_2	-	Histamine 2 receptor
G	-	Gastrin receptors.
PG	-	Prostaglandin receptors.

ACh stimulates M receptors and also induces histamine release from mast cells. Gastrin stimulates G receptor and also induces histamine release from mast cells. Histamine stimulates H_2 receptors.

Stimulation of M or H_2 or G receptors stimulate the parietal cell. This activates enzyme $H^+ K^+$ ATPase, which brings H^+ in GI lumen and sends K^+ inside the cells. This works as proton pump. H^+ in lumen combines with Cl^- and forms HCl. Stimulation of PG receptors inhibit acid secretion.

Acid and pepsin damage gastric mucosa while mucus and bicarbonate protect it.

Acid peptic disorders

These disorders are characterized by increased acid or pepsin secretion. Actually, it is the imbalance between harmful factors (acid, pepsin) for GI mucosa and protective factors (mucus and bicarbonates). Peptic ulcer, GERD, Zollinger Ellison syndrome (ZE syndrome), gastritis etc. are acid peptic disorders

Three important classes of drugs are widely used in all these disorders

i) Antacids
ii) H_2 receptor antagonists
iii) Proton pump inhibitors

ANTACIDS

Antacids are alkalies. They neutralize acid in GI tract and provide pain relief. Antacids are of two types:

i) Systemic antacids: They are absorbed in the blood and cause systemic alkalosis.

ii) Locally acting antacids: They are not (or very poorly) absorbed and act in GI lumen. They are called as nonsystemic antacids.

Antacids neutralize acid and provide temporary relief.

Figure 5.2 Antacids

Antacids

Systemic antacids	Nonsystemic antacids
Sodium bicarbonate	Aluminium hydroxide
Sodium citrate	Aluminium trisilicate
	Magnesium hydroxide (milk of magnesia)
	Magnesium trisilicate
	Magnesium carbonate
	Magaldrate: Hydromagnesium aluminate
	Calcium carbonate.

Mechanism of action

Antacids are alkaline in nature
→ Neutralize acid in stomach
→ Increased pH
→ Pepsin is inactivated in higher pH.

Pepsin is inactivated in higher pH.

Thus, these drugs reduce acid and pepsin and provide pain relief. Antacids act for around 1 hour after administration. Co-administration with food increases duration of action of these agents. Increase in tone of lower esophageal sphincter due to these agents reduces reflux of acid in esophagus. In higher dose they help in healing of ulcers.

Antacids increase tone of lower esophageal sphincter.

Addition of alginic acid to antacids improves the attachment of antacids to mucosal cells and form a frothy layer on gastric contents. Addition of dimethicone or simethicone or methylpolysyloxane reduces surface tension and small bubbles of froth are converted into large bubble and are easily passed. This reduces flatulence, a common side effect with antacids. Sometimes surface anesthetics like oxethazaine are added in antacids.

Alginic acid and defoaming agents are added in antacid formulations

Indications

i) Hyperacidity

ii) Gastritis

iii) Gastric or duodenal ulcer

iv) Zollinger Ellison (ZE) syndrome: It is a tumor of pancreas or duodenum that produces gastric acid hypersecretion.

v) Gastroesophageal reflux: In this condition contents from stomach enter into esophagus and acid in that damages esophageal mucus membrane

All these conditions are characterized by increased acid secretion and antacids provide prompt pain relief.

Systemic antacids are used in metabolic acidosis or to make urine alkaline.

Adverse effects

GI disturbances like diarrhea, constipation, flatulence are common with nonsystemic antacids. Systemic antacids containing Na, cause increased sodium and fluid overload and are responsible for development of edema and are usually avoided, especially in renal and cardiac patients.

Precautions and interactions

1) Antacids reduce absorption of phosphates, ranitidine, digoxin, iron etc.
2) Antacids reduce adsorption of fat soluble vitamins.

Effectivity of individual agents depends on acids neutralizing capacity. The agents are differentiated and combined due to their effects and adverse effects.

Table 5.1 Antacids

Individual agents	Features
Aluminium containing antacids	Produce constipation and have sustained action.
Magnesium containing antacids	Produce diarrhea and have prompt action.
Magnesium hydroxide	Produces diarrhea and have prompt action. Systemic toxicity is present only in renal disorders
Magaldrate: hydroxy magnesium aluminate	Rapid and long acting agent with lesser GI side effects.
Sodium bicarbonate	Systemic antacid. Avoided in gastric conditions. Used in metabolic acidosis.
Calcium carbonate	Calcium containing antacids are also avoided due to their side effects like GI disturbance, hypercalcemia, increased gastrin secretion, etc.

Combinations of antacids containing aluminium and magnesium improve effects and reduce side effects.

Systemic antacids are useful in nongastric indications.

Combination of two antacids, one containing aluminium and the other magnesium, produces prompt and sustained effect. Additionally, diarrhea due to magnesium is compensated by constipation of the other.

Addition of alginic acid or dimethicone produces improved activity and reduce side effects.

Combinations

GELUSIL capsule	:	Dried aluminium hydroxide gel 250 mg Magnesium trisilicate 500 mg
ALLUJEL Suspension	:	Dried aluminium hydroxide gel 400 mg Magnesium hydroxide 400 mg Methylpolysiloxane 30 mg

Status

Antacids are the first line agents in the symptomatic management of acid peptic disorders. They relieve pain immediately but do not prevent acid secretion. These agents are usually used in combination and nonsystemic agents are preferred. They are usually given along with H_2 receptor antagonists.

H_2 RECEPTOR ANTAGONISTS

This is the most widely used class of drugs in management of acid peptic disorders. H_2 blockers do not neutralize the acid that is already secreted but they prevent further acid secretion. Ex. Cimetidine, ranitidine, famotidine, nizatidine

Mechanism of action: (Refer figure 5.1).

These agents block H_2 receptors on parietal cells. Histamine, therefore, does not stimulate parietal cell and H^+ ions are not released in the lumen. It prevents formation of acid in stomach. Additionally, these drugs reduce pepsin secretion.

Pharmacokinetics

These agents can be given orally or by injectable route. Cimetidine undergoes first pass effect and also has got inhibitory action on hepatic microsomal enzymes. These agents are excreted in urine and bile.

H_2 receptor antagonists do not neutralize acid that is already secreted, they prevent secretion of acid.

Indications

Hyperacidity and gastritis: In both these indications, short-term therapy with H_2 blockers is sufficient.

Gastric and duodenal ulcers: H_2 blockers are mainstay in management of peptic ulcer. Prolonged suppression of acid and pepsin secretion help in preventing pain and in healing of ulcers.

Gastroesophageal reflux: Prevention of acid secretion by these agents reduces number of refluxes and prevents subsequent damage to esophagus.

H_2 blockers do not provide immediate pain relief.

ZE-syndrome: These are not drugs of choice but are commonly used to prevent acid secretion.

Preanesthetic medication: H_2 blockers prevent aspiration pneumonia during surgeries by reducing acid secretion.

Allergic rash: Usually allergic response is governed by H_1 receptors on blood vessels. But some times, for total control, H_2 blockade is also essential.

Adverse effects

Headache, giddiness, restlessness, bowel upsets are common side effects with H_2 blockers. Cimetidine has affinity for androgenic receptors and can cause impotence, loss of libido or gynecomastia. It also causes hepatotoxicity.

Precautions and interactions

i) Cimetidine produces rise in serum creatinine levels and used with caution in renal failure

ii) Cimetidine enhances hepatotoxicity of INH and paracetamol

iii) Cimetidine inhibits enzymes required for metabolism of theophylline warfarin, propranolol, etc.

Ranitidine is most commonly used H_2 receptor antagonist. It has fewer side effects and less drug interactions. It is more potent and longer acting.

Table 5.2 H_2 receptor antagonists

Individual agents and dose	Features
Cimetidine 400 mg BD or 800 mg at bed time 200 mg IM or slow IV	Less potent. Side effects more common. Many drug interactions due to microsomal enzyme inhibition. Undergoes first pass effect.
Ranitidine 150 mg BD or 300 mg at bed time (50 mg IM)	More potent and longer acting. Less CNS penetration Less CNS and other side effects. No gynecomastia. No hepatic enzyme inhibition
Famotidine 20 mg BD or 40 mg at bed time	Antagonism is competitive as well as noncompetitive. More potent. Less side effects. No effect on hepatic enzymes.
Roxatidine 75 mg BD 150 mg at bed time	More potent. Less side effects.

Status

These agents are drugs of choice in almost all types of acid peptic disorders (except for ZE syndrome where omeprazole is a choice). These agents reduce acid secretion but do not neutralize acid that is already secreted. Ranitidine is a preferred agent from the class.

PROTON PUMP INHIBITORS

These agents neither neutralize acid that is already secreted nor block any receptors on parietal cells. They inhibit proton pump in parietal cells. The agents include omeprazole, lansoprazole and pantoprazole.

Mechanism of action: (Refer figure 5.1).
Stimulation of parietal cell (by histamine, ACh, or gastrin) activates $H^+ K^+$ ATPase enzyme or proton pump. This activation makes H^+ available in lumen for production of acid. Proton pump inhibitors inhibit H^+K^+ATPase or proton pump and reduce acid formation. As it blocks the final step in the formation of acid, acid secretion caused by stimulation of any receptor (H_2, M or G) is inhibited by these agents.

Omeprazole inhibits enzyme $H^+ K^+$ ATPase and arrests acid secretions for a prolonged period.

Pharmacokinetics
These agents are administered by oral route in enteric coated form as they are degraded at low pH.

Indications: Gastritis, Zollinger-Ellison Syndrome, gastric or duodenal ulcer, gastroesophageal reflux: In all these disorders, proton pump inhibitors reduce acid secretion and prevent pain and help in healing of ulcer. They are drugs of choice in ZE syndrome, gastroesophageal reflux and in all acid peptic disorders resistant to H_2 blockers.

Omeprazole is a drug of choice in ZE syndrome, GERD and in acid peptic disorders that are resistant to H_2 blockers.

Adverse effects
Headache, GI upset and rash are some less serious adverse effects. These agents suppress acid secretion, which reactively causes hypergastrinemia. Omeprazole can cause carcinoid tumor.

Precautions and interactions
1) Omeprazole inhibits hepatic microsomal enzymes and alter actions of benzodiazepines and anticoagulants.
2) Omeprazole is not used in pregnancy and lactation.

Status
In ZE syndrome and severe gastroesophageal reflux, proton pump inhibitors are drugs of choice. In all other acid peptic disorders, they are preferred when H_2 blockers are not effective.

Individual agents
Omeprazole: 20 mg BD or 40 mg OD oral
Lansoprazole: 15-30 mg BD oral

MANAGEMENT OF PEPTIC ULCER

Peptic ulcer is a breech in continuity of mucosa of stomach or duodenum due to imbalance between various secretions that damage and protect mucosa.

Protective secretions	:	Bicarbonates and mucus
Damaging secretions	:	HCl and pepsin.

H.pylori is the organism that plays a crucial role in development of peptic ulcer.

Gastric ulcer: In gastric ulcer, acid secretion is normal and pain is increased after food.

Duodenal ulcer: Acid secretion is usually increased and pain is relieved after food.

Objectives of management

1) Neutralizing acid and relieving pain
2) Prevention of acid secretion
3) Promoting healing of ulcer
4) Prevention of further damage of GI mucosa
5) Eradication of H. pylori bacteria

Nonpharmacological management

1) Regular sleep and feeding habits
2) Avoiding alcohol and smoking
3) Restriction on spicy food
4) Avoiding NSAIDs, (Non Steroidal Antiinflammatory Analgesics), steroids, xanthines, etc. Long term use of these agents causes peptic ulcer.
5) Avoiding stress
6) Bed rest in acute conditions improves healing

Pharmacological management:

Figure 5.3 Drugs used in management of peptic ulcer

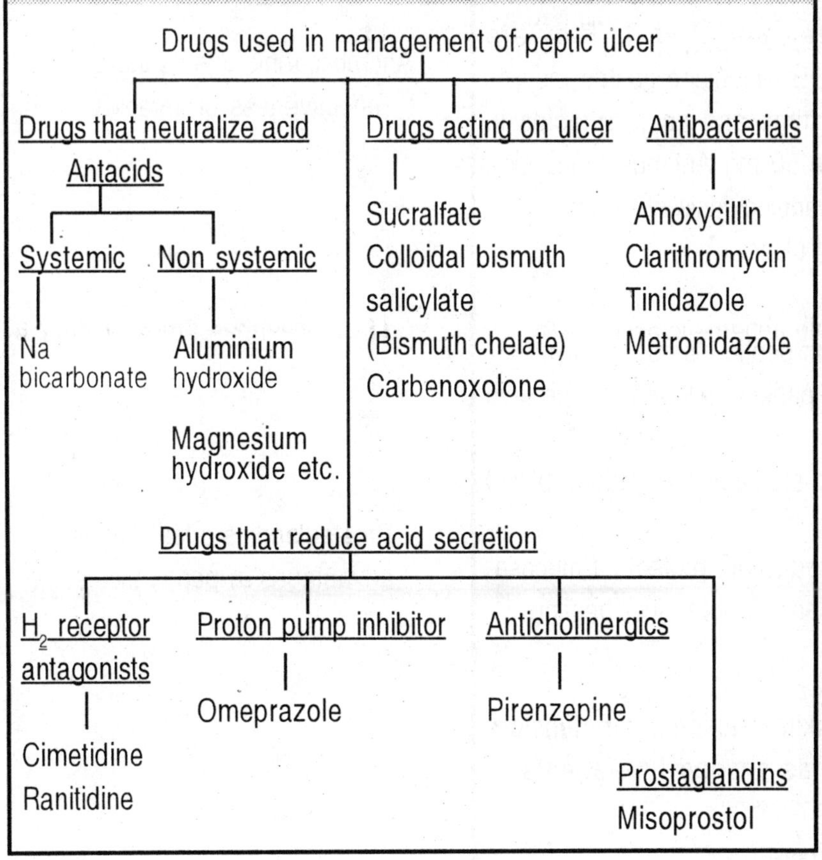

Mechanism by which drugs provide benefits in peptic ulcer:

Antacids: (Refer page 198).

Antacids neutralize the acid in stomach and inactivate pepsin. Both these actions provide pain relief in peptic ulcer. They do not prevent acid secretion and are of symptomatic value only. Nonsystemic antacids are usually preferred to avoid systemic alkalosis. Combinations containing aluminium and magnesium provide prompt and sustained effect and less disturbance in GI motility. Addition of alginic acid to antacids increases adherence of antacids to ulcer and addition of simethicone reduces flatulence.

H_2 receptor antagonists: (Refer page 200).

These drugs block H_2 receptors on parietal cells of stomach and prevent histamine induced acid release. They do not neutralize acid that is already secreted. Hence, they do not provide immediate pain relief. H_2 blockers are drugs of choice for long term management of peptic ulcers. Ex. Ranitidine 300 mg/day OD or 150 mg BD. Cimetidine 400 mg/day OD or 200 mg BD. Ranitidine is preferred due to longer action, more potency, less side effects and less drug interaction.

H_2 blockers are drugs of choice for long term management of peptic ulcers.

Proton pump inhibitors: (Refer page 202).

These drugs inhibit enzyme $H^+ K^+$ ATPase and prevent formation of acid in stomach. In peptic ulcers, they are used in individuals who do not respond to H_2 blockers. Omeprazole - 40 mg/day in single or two doses.

Antimuscarinic agents

These agents block muscarinic receptors on parietal cells of gastric mucosa and reduce ACh mediated release of acid. They are especially useful in nocturnal acidic pain. By inhibiting gastric motility, these agents prolong gastric emptying time and keep antacids in stomach for a long time. Ex. Pirenzepine 50 mg Antimuscarinic side effects like dry mouth, blurred vision, agranulocytosis are rare. These are second line agents in management of ulcer.

Antimuscarinic agents increase effectiveness of antacids.

Prostaglandins: (PGs)

Prostaglandins offer various advantages in peptic ulcers

i) PGs act on prostaglandin receptors on parietal cell and reduce acid secretion. (Refer figure 5.1).

ii) PGs increase bicarbonate secretion in stomach and reduce pH of gastric secretion.

iii) These agents, by increasing mucus production, protect GI mucosa.

iv) They improve gastric cell replication and promote ulcer healing.

vi) They improve circulation of mucosa.

Side effects include GI disturbances, skin reactions, hypotension, uterine bleeding, etc. PGs are used as second line agents in management of ulcers.

Misoprostol 800 μg/day in 3-4 divided doses.

Prostaglandins offer various advantages in peptic ulcers

Sucralfate

It is a complex of sucrose sulfate and aluminium hydroxide. In acidic pH, the complex forms a sticky, viscid, thick gel like polymer that selectively gets attached to the base of ulcer and protects ulcer. Inactivation of acid and bile are additional advantages offered by sucralfate. Sucralfate also increases secretion of mucus. Sucralfate works only in acidic medium, and is not given along with antacids. Side effects: gastric upset, diarrhea, vertigo, sleep disturbances. It is not recommended in pregnancy and in children.

Sucralfate is effective in acidic medium and is not taken along with antacids.

Dose: 1 gm TDS before meal initially. For maintenance: 1 gm OD is sufficient.

Colloidal bismuth salicylate or bismuth chelate

Bismuth chelate stimulates release of prostaglandins, which in turn stimulates secretion of mucus and bicarbonates and protect GI mucosa. This agent chelates protein material in the stomach, forms coat of it on the ulcer base and protects ulcer from acid and pepsin. Detachment of H. pylori from GI mucosa is facilitated by this drug. Darkness of teeth and tongue, nausea, vomiting, etc. are common side effects. Dose: 120 mg TDS before meals.

Detachment of H. pylori from GI mucosa is facilitated by bismuth chelate

Carbenoxolone

Carbenoxolone remains attached to mucosa and increases mucus secretion. It also prolongs life span of gastric epithelial cells and slows their turnover. Reduction in pepsin is another advantage with carbenoxolone. It causes loss of renal potassium and retention of Na and water. Hypokalemia caused by it is dangerous in patients taking cardiac glycosides and Na retention is dangerous in hypertension. Dose 50-100 mg TDS.

Carbenoxolone prolongs life span of gastric epithelial cells and slows their turnover.

Antibacterials

Co-rrelation between H.pylori bacteria and peptic ulcer is now well established. Eradication of H.pylori is an important objective in management of peptic ulcer. Following antibiotics are used for it.

Amoxycillin	500 mg	TDS or 750 mg BD
Clarithromycin	250 mg	BD or 500 mg TDS
Metronidazole	400 mg	TDS or BD
Tinidazole	500 mg	BD
Omeprazole	20 mg	BD
Ranitidine	300 mg	OD

These drugs are used in various combinations like
Amoxycillin + metronidazole + omeprazole or
Amoxycillin + clarithromycin + omeprazole or
Amoxycillin + metronidazole + ranitidine etc.
The treatment, depending on combination, is used for 7 to 15 days.

Management line

Peptic ulcer

↓

Start nonpharmacological management

↓ If not controlled

Start non systemic antacids for symptomatic relief and ranitidine to prevent acid secretion.

↓ If not controlled

Replace ranitidine by omeprazole

↓

Addition of ulcer healing agent depends on individual judgement.

Eradication of H.pylori, if done earlier in the management, is highly helpful. But it is not yet accepted as the first line management.

Eradication of H.pylori, if done earlier in the management, is highly helpful.

Sometimes antianxiety agents provide relief in peptic ulcer.

GASTROESOPHAGEAL REFLUX DISORDER (GERD)

This disease is characterized by reflux of gastric contents into esophagus. They irritate mucosa of esophagus and cause pain (heart burn). Prolonged irritation of mucosa leads to inflammation of esophagus: reflux esophagitis

Objectives of management

i) Pain relief
ii) Reduction in acid secretion
iii) Preventing reflux

Nonpharmacological management

i) Regular feeding habits
ii) No lying down immediately after meals.
iii) Avoiding smoking, alcohol and hot food
iv) Head up position while sleeping

Figure 5.4 Drugs used in the management of GERD

Drugs used in the management of GERD

- Antacids along with alginic acid
- Drugs that prevent acid secretion
  - H_2 blockers: Ranitidine
  - Proton pump inhibitors: Omeprazole
- Prokinetic agents
  - Metoclopramide
  - Cisapride

Mechanism by which drugs act in GERD

1) Antacids (Aluminium hydroxide, magnesium trisilicate, etc.) neutralize acid that is already secreted and reduce pain. Increase in tone of lower esophageal sphincter due to these agents reduces reflux of acid in esophagus.

2) Alginic acid: Alginic acid, when used along with antacids, form frothy coat on the surface of gastric contents and reduces reflux.

3) Ranitidine (300 mg/day in 1,2 doses) by blocking H_2 receptors on parietal cells, reduces secretion of acid. Reflux of less acidic contents causes lesser irritation. Omeprazole (40 mg/day), by inhibiting H^+K^+ATPase enzyme, reduces acid secretion and offers same advantages.

4) Metoclopramide (5-10 mg TDS) and cisapride (10-20 mg TDS) improve gastric emptying and also increase tone of lower esophageal sphincter and reduce reflux.

Metoclopramide and cisapride improve gastric emptying and also increase tono of lower esophageal sphincter and reduce reflux.

Management: Nonpharmacological management is important. Antacids with alginic acid neutralize acid and reduce pain. H_2 blockers are used for long term acid prevention. In resistant cases; omeprazole is the drug of choice. Metoclopramide or cisapride are used simultaneously.

DRUGS USED IN VOMITING

Vomiting: Physiological consideration

Receptors involved in vomiting: dopaminergic, muscarinic, histaminic, 5 hydroxytryptaminergic

Figure 5.5 Physiology of vomiting

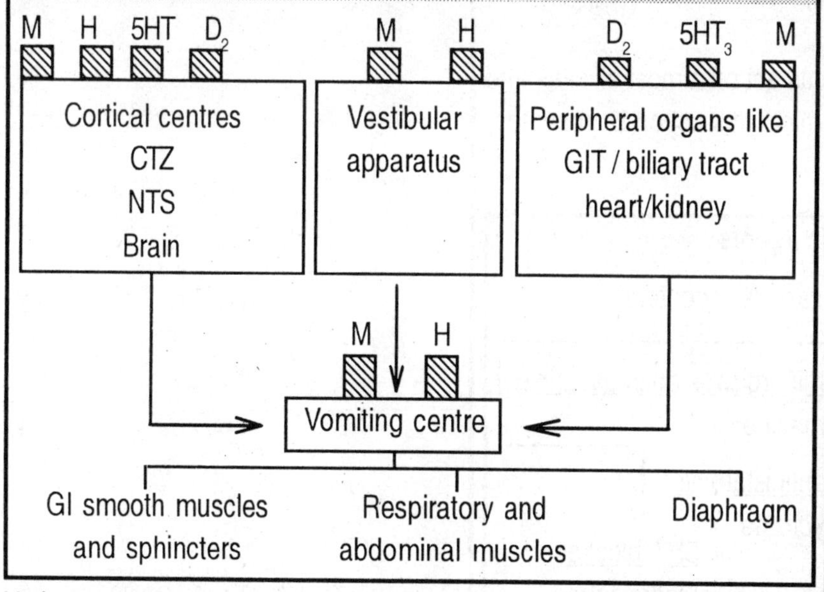

Various causes of vomiting are discussed in 'management of vomiting'

Receptors involved in emesis

CTZ (chemoreceptor trigger zone in brain) and NTS (Nucleus tractus soliterious) contains -

D_2	-	dopaminergic receptors
$5HT_3$	-	5-hydroxytryptamine receptors
M	-	muscarinic receptors
H	-	histaminic receptors.

Vomiting is a forceful expulsion of the products from upper GI tract. It is actually a protective mechanism. Vomiting centre in the medulla coordinates the process of vomiting. It receives stimuli from vestibular apparatus in inner ear, CTZ, NTS and from GI tract, kidney, biliary tract and heart. These organs, when get stimulated by specific stimuli, subsequently stimulate vomiting centre. Vomiting centre when gets stimulated, sends messages to GI smooth muscles, GI sphincters, respiratory and abdominal muscles and diaphragm. All these organs together govern the process of vomiting. Antiperistaltic movements are initiated in stomach and intestine. Abdominal muscles and diaphragm contract and push contents of stomach in esophagus and then out. (Refer figure 5.5).

Vestibular apparatus and vomiting centre contains muscarinic and histaminic receptors. Peripheral organs have dopaminergic, 5HT and muscarinic receptors.

Antiemetic agents

Antiemetic agents prevent vomiting by acting on different receptors. Obviously these agents are blockers of various receptors that are involved in process of vomiting.

I) Antidopaminergics block D_2 receptors in brain and periphery

II) Antihistaminics and antimuscarinics block muscarinic receptors in brain, vestibular apparatus, peripheral organs and vomiting centre.

iii) Anti-5HT agents: They block $5HT_3$ receptors in brain and peripheral organs.

Antihistaminics and antimuscarinics block muscarinic receptors.

Thus, antihistaminic or antimuscarinic agents act on almost all sites and produce antiemetic activity while antidopaminergics act on D_2 receptors in brain and periphery.

Figure 5.6 Antiemetic agents

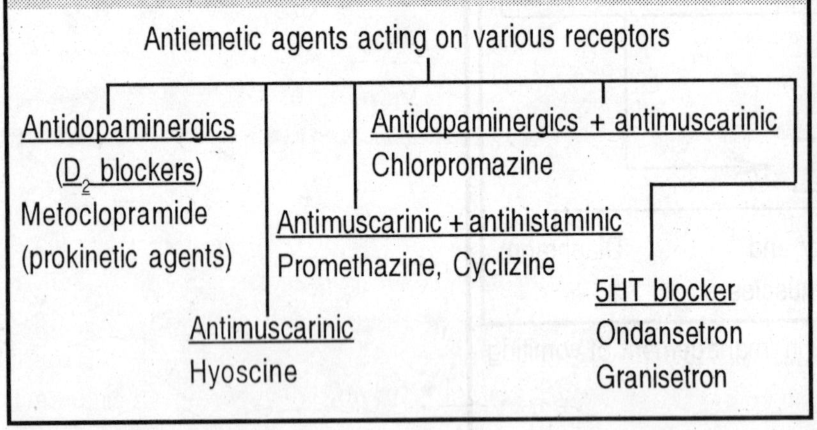

Prokinetic agents

Improvement in peristalsis is referred to as prokinetic action. These agents increase intestinal peristaltic movements and promote gastric emptying. Metoclopramide, domperidone and cisapride are prokinetic agents.

Metoclopramide, domperidone and cisapride are prokinetic agents.

Mechanism of action: (metoclopramide)

Metoclopramide blocks D_2 receptors on CTZ and in gut, blocking of D_2 receptors on CTZ reduce stimulation of CTZ and subsequently that of vomiting centre. This action provides antiemetic effects.

Blocking of D_2 receptors in GI tract increases motility of stomach and intestines. This improves peristalsis. At the same time, tone of lower oesphageal sphincter is increased by it and regurgitation of contents of stomach in oesphagus is prevented.

Metoclopramide enhances release of ACh from nerve endings in GI tract and increases the motility. Metoclopramide has some blocking action on 5HT receptors.

Metoclopramide enhances release of ACh from nerve endings in GI tract and increases the motility.

Indications

1) Nausea and vomiting related to GI disorders: In these conditions, metoclopramide helps due to its central antiemetic actions and peripheral prokinetic actions. Increase in tone of lower oesophageal sphincter also provides additional relief.

2) Metoclopramide also prevents nausea and vomiting associated with migraine, cytotoxic drugs and chemotherapy.

3) Accelerated gastric emptying is required in emergency surgeries or intestinal procedures.

4) Metoclopramide in gastroesophageal reflux provides relief. by (i) improving gastric emptying and (ii) by increasing tone of LES (lower esophageal sphincter).

Table 5.3 Prokinetic agents

Individual agents and dose	Features
Metoclopramide 10 mg TDS oral or IM or 0.5 mg/kg IV children 0.25 to 0.5 mg/kg	Prototype agent
Domperidone 10-40 mg TDS oral children (0.3-0.6 mg / kg)	Less effectivity compared to metoclopramide No action on ACh release. Side effects are less than metoclopramide as it does not cross BBB.
Cisapride 10-20 mg TDS (action is on colon also not by other drugs)	No action on dopaminergic receptors. No antiemetic action. Peripherally (in GI tract) it works by increasing release of ACh. No extrapyramidal side effects or hyperprolactinemia or gynecomastia. Abdominal cramps and diarrhea are common side effects. Cisapride is indicated in gastroesophageal reflux and in constipation. Cardiac arrhythmias are produced when it is used with some antifungal or macrolide agents.

Domperidone has fewer CNS side effects.

Cisapride predominantly acts by enhancing cholinergic action in GI tract.

Adverse effects

Diarrhea, dizziness, extrapyramidal symptoms like facial spasm, trismus restlessness are some side effects of metoclopramide. These effects are mainly present in children and young adults. Long term use may cause gynecomastia or parkinsonism.

MANAGEMENT OF VOMITING

Vomiting is a forceful expulsion of contents of upper GI tract.

Objectives of management

1) Prevention of further attacks of vomiting
2) Fluid and electrolyte replacement
3) Investigating and treating cause

Figure 5.7 Drugs used in vomiting

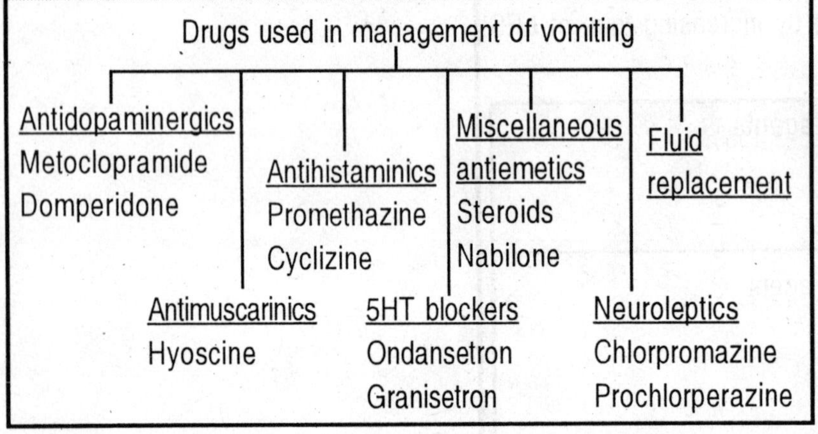

Antidopaminergics: (Refer Page 208).

These drugs act on D_2 receptor in CTZ and GIT and prevent vomiting. Improvement in peristalsis and increase in tone of LES also add to antiemetic action. These are preferred agents in vomiting associated with GI disorders, drug induced vomiting, vomiting in migraine or heart diseases. Ex. Metoclopramide: 10 mg TDS oral or IM

Antimuscarinic agents and antihistaminic agents

Antimuscarinic agents block muscarinic receptor in CTZ, vomiting centre, GI tract and vestibular apparatus. Blocking of receptors from all sites provides complete antiemetic protection. Antihistaminics offers advantages in the same way. Their action is mediated through histaminic as well as muscarinic receptors. These are usually drugs of choice in motion sickness.

Antimuscarinic agent: Hyoscine 0.2-0.4 mg oral or IM or patch of 1.5 mg. Antihistaminic + antimuscarinic agent: promethazine: 25 mg. Sedative action of antihistaminic adds to antiemetic action.

Hyoscine patches are effectively used in motion sickness.

Neuroleptics

They mainly act by blocking D_2 receptors in CTZ but additional blockade of muscarinic receptors on vomiting centre also improves antiemetic activity. They are given in drug induced vomiting, migraine, vomiting associated with liver disorders, in morning sickness, etc. They are usually avoided due to their effects on CNS. Prochlorperazine 5-10 mg TDS or QID, IM. Chlorpromazine 10-25 mg QID, oral or injectable.

5HT antagonists

These agents block 5 HT receptors in peripheral organs and in CTZ and prevent vomiting. These agents are preferred in radiation and drug induced vomiting. They are also effectively used in vomiting associated with GI, liver or biliary disorders and in post operative nausea and vomiting. Headache and constipation are common side effects. Dose: Ondansetron 8 - 32 mg IV infused over 15 minutes, (half an hour before starting cancer chemotherapy). It can be given in oral form in doses of 8 mg TDS. It is also used preoperatively. Granisetron: 1 mg BD

Additional agents

Corticosteroids like dexamethasone, methylprednisolone or benzodiazepine like lorazepam are used as adjuvants to antiemetic agents. Nabilone is a synthetic cannabinoid that is used along with standard antiemetic agents. It is preferred in vomiting that is resistant to standard drugs. It is especially useful in vomiting associated with cancer chemotherapy.

Fluid and electrolyte replacement must be done promptly in case of vomiting that leads to dehydration.

Management line

There is no standard line of management for vomiting. Drug of choice depends on cause of vomiting.

Drug of choice in vomiting depends on the cause.

i) Motion sickness: It is the disorder characterized by nausea and vomiting due to body motion. Vestibular apparatus is involved in pathophysiology of motion sickness. In case of severe motion sickness journey must be discontinued. Prophylactically hyoscine (oral or patch) is the drug of choice. Alternatively, promethazine is used. These agents are best useful if taken an hour before journey.

ii) For drug or radiation induced vomiting and pre and post operative nausea and vomiting, Ondansetron or metoclopramide can be used. Chlorpromazine is also effective but rarely used due to side effects.

iii) Morning sickness is the nausea and vomiting in pregnancy due to hormonal imbalance. It usually gets resolved after 3 months of pregnancy. Many times only assurance is enough. If drugs are required, prochlorperazine can be used effectively. Drugs like pyridoxine, cyclizine or metoclopramide are helpful in certain cases.

Use of antiemetic drugs in pregnancy should be discouraged

iv) In vomiting, associated with peripheral disorders like GI disorders, heart or renal disorders, biliary stones etc., ondansetron or metoclopramide is used.

In severe vomiting, fluid and electrolyte replacement is a crucial part in management.

DIARRHOEA

Diarrhoea is a frequent passage of poorly formed stools. Water and electrolyte loss during diarrhea is a major reason for morbidity and mortality in India.

Pathophysiology: Diarrhoea is caused by a variety of reasons.

1) Infective diarrhoea: Organism like protozoa, bacteria, viruses invade and irritate GI mucosa. Attempt to remove those organisms by body, result in increased motility and secretions. Water, Na chlorides, bicarbonates are lost in diarrhea. Traveller's diarrhea is usually due to mixed infections or by any of these organisms. Diarrhea in AIDS is also due to superinfection or sometimes it is drug induced.

2) Ulcerative colitis: Ulcerative colitis is characterized by large ulcerations and inflammed areas in intestines. This can be due to allergic reactions, bacterial infections or due to autoimmune reactions. It leads to increased secretion of bicarbonates and then sodium.

3) Drug induced diarrhoea: Many drugs cause diarrhea as side effects. Ex. Antibiotics like tetracycline, ampicillin, sorbitol, magnesium containing antacids.

4) Psychogenic diarrhoea: Emotional disturbances lead to parasympathetic stimulation. It results in excess secretion of mucus and some electrolytes. Stool content may not increase every time. Increased motility of intestines contribute to diarrheal attack.

5) Spurious diarrhoea: Use of purgatives in constipation, some times only stimulates secretions which are passed without relieving the constipation.

6) Pancreatic insufficiency or lactose intolerance cause osmotic entry of fluids in intestines and induce diarrhea.

Fluid and electrolyte loss is associated with almost all types of diarrhea and their replacement is the first step in management of diarrhea. Loss of fluid and electrolytes result in dehydration, hypovolemic shock, metabolic acidosis and death.

Fluid and electrolyte replacement in diarrhoea

Fluids and electrolytes lost in diarrhea can be replaced, by oral or intravenous route depending on condition of the patient. ORS: Oral rehydration solution is the solution designed by WHO to compensate fluid loss during diarrhoea.

Content	Amount in gm
NaCl	3.5
KCl	1.5
Na citrate	2.9
Anhydrous glucose	20

It is taken in 1 litre of water. It provides Na^+ 90 mM, K^+ 20 mM, Cl^- 80 mM. Citrate 30 mM and glucose 110 mM. Some variations are also present in this formula. Formula for infants contains less amount of Na or another WHO formula contains $NaHCO_3$ in place of Na citrate. (But $NaHCO_3$ forms brown coloration with glucose and not commonly used).

Fluid and electrolyte replacement is the most important aspect in management of diarrhea.

Cereal based ORS

Though glucose based ORS solutions replace fluid and electrolytes, they do not reduce stool volume. (In fact sometimes increase it). Boiled rice powder (40-50 g/lit) is a good substitute for glucose. It reduces stool volume and duration of disease. It acts by directly inhibiting chloride channels. Proteins in rice stimulate salt and water absorption.

Cereal based ORS reduces stool volume.

Mechanism of action

The formulation is taken in one litre water. This supplies fluid support. Glucose facilitates transport of Na in cells. All other components compensate the quantity of electrolytes lost.

Potentiating the action of ORS: Glycine or alanine like amino acids are some times added in ORS. These amino acids improve active transport of Na in the body.

Indications: ORS is used in any condition in which fluid loss is <10% of body weight. ORS is used in diarrheas, dehydration due to burns or trauma and in post-surgical cases.

Status: ORS is the first line therapy and life saving medication in dehydration.

Intravenous fluid therapy

Intravenous fluid replacement is indicated when:

i) Total fluid loss is more than 10% of body weight,

ii) Vomiting does not permit oral fluid replacement,

iii) Patient is weak or not in conscious state to take ORS.

Total fluid loss, if is more than 10% of body weight, IV fluid replacement is required.

The composition usually is

5 gm NaCl;

1 gm KCl;

4 gm $NaHCO_3$ in 1 liter water or 5% glucose saline.

This provides 133 mM Na^+, 13 mM K^+, 98 mM Cl^-, and 48 mM HCO_3^-.

Management of diarrhoea

Diarrhea is a frequent passage of loosely formed stools. It needs fluid replacement immediately. Requirement of curative treatment depends on the cause of diarrhea.

Objectives of management

1) Fluid and electrolyte replacement
2) Nutritional supplements
3) Preventing diarrheal attacks
4) Treatment of the cause

Nonpharmacological management

Sufficient amount of water

Rice in diet breaks down into amino acids and glucose in intestines and improve transport of Na and water in the body.

Commercial soft drinks do not contain sufficient Na and so they are not of much help.

Banana, citrus fruits, coconut water, rice should contain major part of diet.

Fibres, pulses, fried food should be avoided

Rice containing diet is helpful in diarrhea

Figure 5.8 Drugs used in diarrhoea

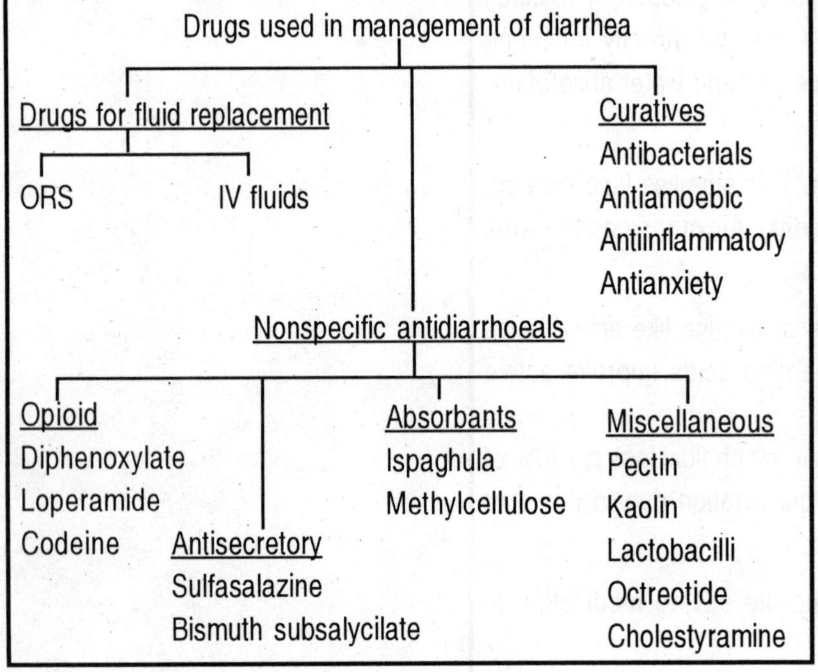

Mechanism by which drugs act in diarrhoeas

1) ORS or intravenous fluids: (Refer page 212).

These agents replace fluid and electrolytes that are lost in diarrheal attacks. These are life saving drugs and they are used as the first line management. Details of fluid replacement therapy are already discussed.

2) Opioids

In diarrhea, opioids act by central and peripheral mechanisms. They act on opioid receptor and:

i) Reduce GI motility,

ii) Reduce amount of secretions,

iii) Improve tone of GI sphincters,

iv) Promote reabsorption of Na and water.

Antimotility agents inhibit removal of pathogens from GI tract.

Constipation, toxic megacolon, CNS alterations, respiratory depression are the common adverse effects with opioids. Diphenoxylate (2.5-20 mg/day) and loperamide (2 - 16 mg/day) are commonly used agents. To avoid misuse of opioids, atropine is combined in low dose in antidiarrheal formulations (Lomotil contains diphenoxylate and atropine). Adverse effects of atropine (like dry mouth or blurring of vision) reduce misuse of opioids. These agents are usually avoided in infectious diarrhea and ulcerative colitis. Codeine: 15-60 mg TDS.

3) Sulfasalazine: It is 5-aminosalicylic acid compound. It reduces formation of prostaglandins. Inhibition of PGs results in reduced secretions in GI tract and control over diarrheas. Additional advantage is antiinflammatory activity that is offered due to inhibition of PGs. Dose: (0.5-2 mg) Mesalamine is similar type of drug, which can be given by oral route (400 mg) or by enema. These agents are preferred in diarrhea of inflammatory origin. GI disturbances, rash, joint pains, headache are common side effects.

4) Bismuth subsalicylate acts by reducing PG synthesis (which in turn reduces GI secretions). It also adsorbs bacterial toxins. It is helpful in infectious diarrheas. (262 mg)

Sulfasalazine is preferred in inflammatory diarrhea, Bismuth subsalycilate in infectious diarrhea and octreotide in secretory diarrhea.

5) Octreotide: It is analogue of somatostatin. It reduces secretion of gastric acid, pepsinogen, bicarbonates, VIP and cholecystokinins. It also inhibits intestinal contractions. It is mainly used in secretory diarrheas associated with insulinoma, glucagonoma, carcinoid tumor etc.

6) Lactobacilli: These are organisms from natural flora of GI tract. If they are administered externally, they maintain normal flora of GI and prevent growth of pathogens and prevent diarrhea.

7) Cholestyramine: It is anion exchange resin. It inactivates bile salts and reduces colonic irritation (12-24 gm oral).

8) Ispaghula and methyl cellulose absorb fluids in GI tract and reduce urgencies.

9) Kaolin probably adsorbs water, bile, bacteria and bacterial toxins. (2-4 gm oral QID)

10) Pectin helps in formation of solid stools

Management line

1) Immediate fluid replacement

If fluid loss < 10% of Body weight - use ORS

If fluid loss > 10% of Body weight or ORS administration not possible due to vomiting and unconsciousness: use IV fluids.

Use of nonspecific antimotility antidiarrheals should be discouraged

2) Use of nonspecific antimotility - antidiarrheal agents is done only when it is very essential (like important day to day activities or travelling). The reduced passage of stools by these drugs may accumulate pathogens in GI tract.

Nonspecific antidiarrheal: loperamide, diphenoxylate

3) Supportive antidiarrheals

Sulfasalazine in diarrhea of inflammatory origin.

Bismuth subsalicylate: in infectious diarrhea

Octreotide in secretory diarrheas.

4) Treatment of cause

Antiinfective agents: Use of these agents in diarrhea is a sensitive and controversial issue. Routinely, investigations are not done to confirm the causative organisms. Infectious diarrhea many times is self limiting. Depending on the situation, antiprotozoals like metronidazole, tinidazole and antibacterials like ciprofloxacin, norfloxacin are used in diarrheas.

Routinely, investigations are not done to confirm the causative organisms.

Drug induced diarrhea: Decision in this situation depends on the drug causing diarrhea. Dose of the drug is reduced or alternative agent is used if possible. Diarrheas due to anxiety and ulcerative colitis are treated with antiinflammatory or antianxiety agents.

CONSTIPATION

Constipation is infrequent production of hard stools that require straining. Consistency of stools usually governs the frequency of stools and efforts that are required to pass the stools. Water content of stools decides the consistency. In a way, it is the water content that governs the passage of stools. Reduction in water content of stool is responsible for constipation.

Inadequate fluid intake, reduced fibres in diet, lack of exercise, irregularities in bowel habits, painful defecation (in piles or fissures) are some of the causes of constipation. Long term constipation and straining during defecation can lead to piles, fissures, cardiac strain, headache. Hence proper treatment of constipation is essential.

Consequences of constipation are hardly benign.

Management of constipation

Objectives

i) To increase water content of stools
ii) To reduce strain while passing stools
iii) To prevent complications of constipation

Nonpharmacological management

Increase in water intake
Diet containing fibres e.g. carrot, beat, green leafy vegetables
Regular bowel habits
Exercise
Psychological assurance
All these factors can relieve constipation without drug therapy

Drugs used in management of constipation

Drugs that are used in constipation are called as laxatives (or purgatives, evacuants, aperients, or cathartics). Though these terms are used interchangeably: laxative is the term used for drugs that form semisolid stools and purgative or cathartics are the terms for drugs that form liquid stools.

Pharmacological management

Various drugs are used for the treatment of constipation. Pharmacological treatment should be supported by nonpharmacological measures.

Figure 5.9 Laxatives

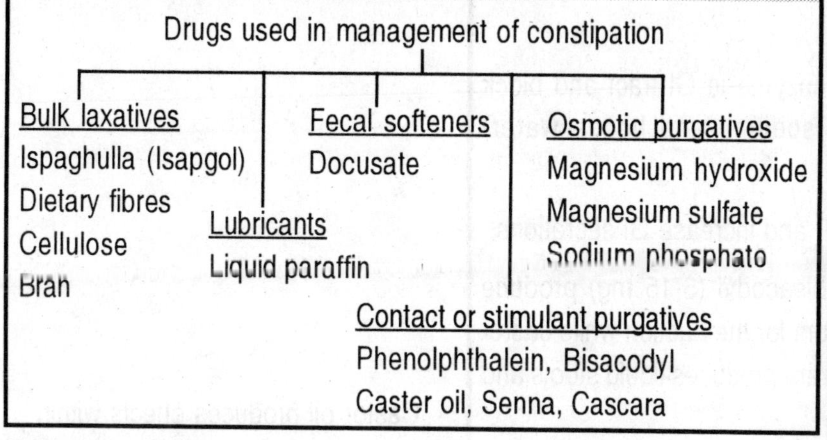

Bulk laxatives

These agents, after oral administration, are not broken down by enzymes and are not absorbed. When taken along with water, they absorb water, swell and increase volume of stools and make stools soft. Increase in volume of stools stimulates physiological reflex bowel activity and there is almost a natural passage of stools.

> Bulk laxatives stimulate physiological reflex bowel activity. They must be taken with water.

Bulk laxatives take 1-3 days for their action. Side effects of bulk laxatives are rare but administration of large quantities and palatability are limiting factors. In addition to constipation, these agents are used to reduce appetite and to reduce cholesterol.

> Bulk laxatives are best but they take time.

Ispaghulla is the most widely used agents. Methyl cellulose or psyllium are alternative agents from this class.

Status: Due to physiological action, bulk laxatives are the safest and the ideal agents.

Lubricants: Liquid paraffin

This petroleum hydrocarbon is a chemically inert mineral oil. It is not digested after oral administration. It reduces absorption of water from intestines and increases the water content of stools. Additionally paraffin, due to its oily properties, makes stools soft and reduces friction of stools with the intestinal walls .

Disadvantages with liquid paraffin include: unpleasant taste, lipoid pneumonia due to aspiration into respiratory tract, leakage through anal canal, reduced absorption of fat soluble vitamins, etc.
Paraffin takes 8-12 hours to produce effects. Dose is 15-30 ml per day

Fecal softener: Docusate

Docusate lowers surface tension of water in stools, due to which more amount of water is retained in the stools and stools become soft. Its action on GI mucosa also increase water content in the lumen. It takes 1-2 days to produce action. Dose 100-200 mg.

Contact or stimulant purgatives

These agents that produce semisolid or liquid stools are called as purgatives. They produce purgative effects by different mechanism:

1) They stimulate sensory nerve endings in GI mucosa or mesenteric plexus and increase motility of GI tract.

2) These agents inhibit Na^+ K^+ ATPase enzyme in GI tract and block absorption of sodium. This increases sodium (and hence water) content in lumen.

3) They stimulate formation of cyclic AMP and increase GI secretions.

Agents: Phenolphthalein (60-130 mg) bisacodyl (5-15 mg) produce semisolid stools and take around 8-10 hours for their action while caster oil (15-20 ml in adults and 5-15 ml in children) produces liquid stools and takes 2-6 hours for action.

Castor oil produces effects within 2 - 6 hours.

Fluid and electrolyte imbalance, cramps, atony, abortions are side effects that are reported with these agents. Cascara, senna are some additional contact purgatives.

Osmotic purgatives: (Saline purgatives)

As the name suggests, these are osmotically active substances. Due to their osmotic activity they retain water in intestines and increase water content of stools. They are fast acting, require 2-4 hours for their action, and produce watery stools. They are not routinely used for constipation but preferred for emptying bowel before surgeries and after treatment for worms. Ex. Magnesium sulfate (more effective), magnesium hydroxide (less effective), sodium sulfate etc.

Osmotic laxatives are not preferred for constipation but are used to empty GI tract before surgical procedures.

Lactulose: This osmotic purgative has 3 actions (1) It is a disaccharide and is not digested; hence retains water. (2) It breaks down into osmotically active substances and retains water due to osmotic activitiy. (3) It reduces growth of colonic organisms that produce ammonia. This action is helpful in liver disorders or in encephalopathies where nitrogenous substances are excess in the body. It requires 1-2 days for laxative effects. Dose up to 60 mg/day.

Lactulose reduces growth of colonic organisms.

Management line for constipation

Initially constipation must be treated with nonpharmacological management. If it is not effective, bulk laxatives should be the drugs of choice. Lubricants or stool softeners are used in resistant cases. In elderly population, where straining is a problem, lubricants are preferred. Contact or stimulant laxatives should be used as a last choice. But they can be preferred in spastic constipation.

Prolonged or continuous use of laxatives should be discouraged as it can cause laxative abuse. Laxatives are avoided in presence of intestinal obstructions. In pregnancy, as far as possible, laxatives are avoided. They can induce abortion. In case of drug induced constipation, the constipating drug (opioids, NSAIDs, antidiarrheals, aluminium containing antacids, etc.) is either substituted with other agents

Laxatives are not used in intestinal obstruction.

or dose adjustment is done. If this is not possible, short-term use of bulk laxatives or nonpharmacological management is sufficient.

Other indications for laxatives or purgatives

1) Saline purgatives or stimulants are used for emptying bowels before investigative procedures and surgeries.

2) To avoid strain, bulk laxatives are administered prophylactically in bed ridden patient, in cardiac patients or in patients of piles or fissures. If not effective, lubricants or contact laxatives are used.

3) After deworming, osmotic laxatives are used to flush out worms and drug.

4) Saline purgatives are used in oral poisoning to remove the poison in the GI tract.

Laxative abuse

Abuse is unindicated use of drugs to get pleasure. Compared to normal defecation, laxatives offer more complete evacuation of intestines and so extra sense of pleasure. Hence, once they are used, there is a desire to repeat them without any medical indication. Initially this dependence is psychological, then it gets converted into physical dependence.

Disadvantages of laxative abuse

i) GI disturbances like flatulence, nausea, anorexia, etc.
ii) No defecation without laxatives
iii) Water and electrolyte depletion
iv) Intestinal rupture is possible if purgatives are taken in presence of obstruction.
v) Malabsorption: Laxatives interfere in absorption of all nutrients including vitamins and minerals.
vi) Irritable bowel syndrome

Laxatives interfere in absorption of all nutrients including vitamins and minerals.

The treatment for laxative abuse highly depends on doctor's assurance and patient's clarification about concept of constipation. It must be clarified to the patient that the reduction in frequency is not the only criteria for constipation. Regular bowel habits, plenty of water, fibrous diet, exercises and gradual withdrawal of laxatives can reduce dependence.

DIGESTANTS

Digestants are the substances that potentiate the process of digestion. These agents are used when there is deficiency of natural digestants.

Table 5.4 Digestants

Individual agents	Features
Diluted HCl	Increase in appetite. Activation of pepsin.
Pepsin, papain, renin	Digestion of proteins.
Pancreatin or pancrealipase (It contains amylase, lipase, trypsin)	Digestion of carbohydrates, proteins and lipid. Proteins, in presence of pancreatin, are digested even in absence of gastric enzymes.
Taka diastase	Digestion of carbohydrates.

Bile salts, bile acids and cheno-deoxycholic acids (CDCA) are ingredients in bile and primarily are involved in digestion of fats. CDCA also increases secretion of bile. It is also used to dissolve gall stone.

Indications of digestants

i) Chronic gastrointestinal problems in which digestion is hampered

ii) Reduced HCl secretion in stomach, achlorhydria

iii) Pancreatic insufficiency or liver disorders

iv) Gastrectomy and pancreaectomy

CARMINATIVES

Carminatives reduce flatulence. These agents irritate GI mucosa, induce peristalsis, relax sphincters and facilitate expulsion of gases and reduce discomfort.

Table 5.5 Carminatives

Individual agents	Features
Sodium bicarbonate (Gripe waters)	It stimulates production of CO_2, which causes distension of stomach and promotes expulsion of gases through eructation.
Methylpolysiloxane	It is an antifoaming agent. It converts small air bubbles into large by reducing surface tension and makes passage of gases easy.
Ginger/peppermint	These agents are irritants. They dilate lower esophageal sphincter and promote expulsion of gases.

Indications: Flatulence, indigestion, postprandial epigastric tightness, preoperative preparation, postoperative gastric discomfort, etc.

EMETICS

Emetic agents induce vomiting. Vomiting actually is a reflex that protects GI tract from harmful substances. In poisoning, emesis is induced to prevent further absorption of poison. Depending on their actions emetic agents are divided into three groups.

Figure 5.10 Emetics

Emetics

- Acting on GI tract → Salt, mustard
- Acting on CTZ → Apomorphine
- Acting on both CTZ and GI tract → Ipecac

Table 5.6 Emetics

Individual agent	Features
1) Salt and mustard (oral)	Cause strong irritation of GI tract and induce vomiting. Taken along with plenty of water.
2) Apomorphine (injectable) SC or IM	Stimulates D_2 receptors on CTZ and induces vomiting in 3-5 minutes. Not given orally.
3) Ipecac syrup	Acts as GI irritant and also stimulates CTZ. Taken along with water. It takes 15-20 minutes for action. If there is no effect, repeated doses are administered.

Indication

Emetics are used to induce expulsion of orally administered poisons to prevent further absorption

Contraindications: Emetics are not given in:

i) Unconscious or semiconscious patient: In these patients emesis can cause aspiration pneumonia due to entry of GI contents into respiratory tract.

ii) Corrosive poisoning: These poison can cause esophageal perforations.

iii) Petroleum poisons: Aspiration pneumonia is common during vomiting of petroleum poisons.

DRUGS IN RESPIRATORY SYSTEM

"THIS SECTION CONTAINS"

TOXICOLOGY

METHYL XANTHINES

Theophylline, theobromine and caffeine are three naturally occurring xanthines. Tea, coffee and cocoa are natural sources of methyl xanthines. Aminophylline or choline theophyllinates are the derivatives of theophylline. Caffeine and theophylline are potent methyl xanthines while theobromine is weak.

Caffeine and theophylline are potent methyl xanthines.

Mechanism of action

1) These agents block adenosine receptors situated on various organs and prevent adenosine mediated stimulation of these receptors. It is the most predominant action that produces bronchodilatation.

Methyl xanthines block adenosine receptors.

2) Xanthines inhibit phosphodiesterase enzyme. This enzyme converts cyclic AMP into 5-AMP and cyclic GMP into 5-GMP. Inhibition of this enzyme results in accumulation of cGMP and cAMP, which in turn produces bronchodilatation, vasodilatation and cardiac stimulation.

Xanthines inhibit phosphodiesterase enzyme.

3) Xanthines release Ca from sarcoplasmic reticulum and improve contraction of skeletal and cardiac muscles.

Pharmacological actions

i) Bronchodilatation

ii) Stimulation of myocardium: ↑ force of contraction and heart rate, stimulation of vasomotor centre and transient vasodilatation are the actions of xanthines on CVS. The net result is cardiac stimulation and rise in BP but effects are variable.

iii) Thiazide like diuretic action: weak diuresis

vi) Improvement in performance of skeletal muscles by xanthines provides additional advantage in bronchial asthma.

v) Xanthines increase acid and pepsin secretion in stomach.

vi) These agents can stabilize mast cells and prevent release of allergic mediators.

vii) CNS actions: Stimulation of mental activities, increased physical and skill performance, improved alertness and wakefulness, postponement of sleep and boredom.

Pharmacokinetics

Theophylline is well absorbed orally. The peculiar feature in kinetics is that after certain dose it follows zero order kinetics. (Refer page 24). This increases the accumulation of drug in the body. As the therapeutic range of it is narrow, slight increase in concentration can increase the magnitude of effects and side effects in large proportion. This fact has limited the use of these agents in practice.

Therapeutic range of theophylline is narrow.

Indications

1) Bronchial asthma: xanthines offer following advantages in bronchial asthma.

i) Bronchodilatation

ii) Improved mucocilliary clearance of respiratory secretion.

iii) Improved ventilatory efforts by action on respiratory centre.

iv) Mast cell stabilization (it reduces release of allergic mediators from mast cells).

2) Neonatal apnea: These agents offer prompt bronchodilatation.

3) Analgesic adjuvant: Caffeine is used to potentiate analgesic effects of nonsteroidal antiinflammatory drugs or ergots in migraine.

Caffeine is used with nonsteroidal antiinflammatory drugs.

Adverse effects:

These agents have narrow therapeutic range and adverse effects are very common: Gastric discomfort, diarrhea, pain in abdomen, anxiety restlessness, tremors, confusion, hypotension, etc.

Acute IV toxicity causes hypotension, convulsions, arrhythmias and sudden death.

Table 6.1 Methyl xanthines

Individual agents and dose	Features
Theophylline (anhydrous) 100 - 300 mg TDS	Predominant action on lungs and heart.
Aminophylline 250 mg oral or IV in glucose saline	Derivative of theophylline Highly soluble
Etophylline 250 mg oral, IV, IM	Derivative of theophylline
Choline theophyllinate 500 mg oral	
Caffeine	Major action is on CNS and skeletal muscles

Precautions and interactions

They are used with caution in pregnancy and lactation.

These drugs increase acid secretion and are taken along with food.

Therapeutic drug monitoring is required in crucial cases.

Pulse rate and BP must be watched during IV infusion.

Theophylline metabolism is increased by phenytoin, barbiturates smoking, alcohol, etc.

Theophylline metabolism is inhibited by H_2 receptor antagonists and OC pills.

Pulse rate and BP must be watched during IV infusion.

Status

Due to narrow therapeutic range these agents are not used as first line agents in bronchial asthma. In refractory cases and in severe attacks xanthines are used by oral or IV route.

MAST CELL STABILIZERS

Physiological considerations

Antigen-antibody reactions stimulate mast cells. Mast cells in the body, when are stimulated, release various allergic and inflammatory mediators like histamine, PAF, (platelet activating factor), leukotrienes etc.

Mast cell stabilizers prevent release of these mediators from mast cells. These agents include sodium cromoglycate or cromolyn sodium, nedocromil and ketotifen.

Mechanism of action

These agents prevent degranulation of mast cells and inhibit subsequent release of mediators involved in process of allergy and inflammation. They do not have any effects on bronchi that are already constricted.

These agents prevent degranulation of mast cells.

Indications

These agents are used in bronchial asthma to prevent release of mediators involved in bronchial asthma. They are especially useful in exercise induced asthma. They relieve respiratory symptoms and reduce dose of bronchodilators. They are also used in conjunctivitis and stomatitis.

Side effects

Headache, throat irritation, dizziness, rash, etc.

Table 6.2 Mast cell stabilizers

Individual agents and dose	Features
Disodium cromoglycate 1 mg / dose 2 puffs QID	Not used orally: spinhalers are used Usually combined with steroids. Trial period is required to asses efficacy of this agent. Side effects are very rare.
Nedocromil sodium 4 mg (2 puffs)	Side effects are more with it.
Ketotifen 1-2 mg BD 0.5 mg BD - Children	Can be used orally Additional antihistaminic and sedative property. Also effective in other allergic conditions like dermatitis, rash etc.

These agents are used as second line agents in bronchial asthma.

Status

These agents are used as second line agents in bronchial asthma. Commonly used along with steroids or some bronchodilators.

MANAGEMENT OF BRONCHIAL ASTHMA

Physiological considerations

Bronchial asthma is increased responsiveness of tracheobronchial tree characterized by airway inflammation and obstruction.

Extrinsic asthma is increased responsiveness to external allergens like dust, mites, animal dandruff, pollens, etc. Intrinsic asthma is not induced by external factors but said to be due to internal allergens.

Prostaglandins, histamine, heparin, TNF, leukotrienes, interleukin and PAF are some mediators involved in mediation of asthma.

Objectives of management of asthma

i) Avoiding exposure to allergens
ii) Symptomatic relief in acute attack
iii) Preventing future attacks
iv) Normal pulmonary function between 2 attacks
v) Searching for antigen.

Nonpharmacological management

Avoiding exposure to extrinsic allergens

Avoiding active and passive smoking

Restriction on citrus fruits, pickles, cold drinks

Drugs like β blockers, NSAIDs, cholinergics, ACE inhibitors should not be used as they can induce asthma.

Deep breathing exercises, relaxation, yoga help in reducing stress. Stress can induce asthma.

Pharmacological management:

Drug intervention is possible at various stages of asthma.

Figure 6.1 Stages of asthma and use of drugs

Pathophysiology	**Intervention**
Allergen	Avoid exposure Drug prophylaxis
Release of mediators	**Inhibiting release of meditors** Sodium cromoglycate, β_2 stimulants (mast cell stabilize action)
Bronchoconstriction	**Bronchodilators** β_2 - stimulants Theophylline
Inflammation	**Antiinflammatory drugs** Steroids
Complications	Oxygen Emergency management

Figure 6.2 Drugs in asthma

Drugs used in management of asthma

- Drugs that reduce release of mediators
  - Mast cell stabilizers
  - Sodium cromoglycate
  - Nedocromil
  - Ketotifen
- Bronchodilators
  - Sympathomimetics
    - Salbutamol
    - Terbutaline
    - Adrenaline
    - Salmeterol
  - Methyl xanthines
    - Theophylline
    - Aminophylline
    - Etophylline
  - Antimuscarinics
    - Ipratropium bromide
- Glucocorticoids
  - Systemic
    - Prednisolone
    - Hydrocortisone
  - Local aerosol
    - Beclomethasone
    - Triamcinolone
    - Budesonide
- Miscellaneous
  - Antihistaminics
  - PAF antagonists
  - Methotrixate, Gold

Mechanisms by which drugs produce effects in bronchial asthma

Sympathomimetic agents: These agents stimulate β_2 receptors on the bronchi and produce bronchodilatation. Salbutamol, terbutaline and salmeterol are preferred agents due to their β_2 selective action. Still adrenaline is also used in some clinical situations. β_2 stimulants also interfere in the release of histamine from mast cells and reduce mucus production.

β_2 selective agents are prefferd in asthma

Salbutamol : 100-200 mcg inhalation or 2-4 mg oral

Terbutaline : 250 mcg inhalation, 5 mg oral 0.25 mg SC

Adrenaline : 3-0.5 ml of 1:1000 or 0.01 ml/kg IV in severe conditions.

Methyl xanthines (Refer page 223)

Methyl xanthines produce bronchodilatation due to their blocking action on adenosine receptors and due to accumulation of cyclic AMP. Additionally they improve mucociliary clearance. Improved ventilatory activity by these agents also contributes in bronchial asthma.

Theophylline 100-300 mg TDS, Aminophylline 250 mg oral or IV in 20-50 ml of glucose over 20 minutes in emergencies.

Anticholinergics: (Refer page 81). Ipratropium bromide blocks muscarinic receptors on bronchi and prevent ACh mediated bronchoconstriction. It is predominantly used in refractory cases as second line agents. Dose: 40-80 mg inhalation.

Mast cell stabilizers: These agents prevent release of allergic and inflammatory mediators from mast cells and prevent attack of asthma. They are not useful in controlling acute attack of asthma. These are also second line agents. Sodium cromoglycate 2 puffs QID or ketotifen 1-2 mg BD

Corticosteroids: Corticosteroids act as antiinflammatory-antiallergic agents and produce relief in asthma. Additionally, these agents improve responsiveness to β stimulants. Dose: Beclomethasone 100-200 mcg inhalation BD-TID. Prednisolone 20-60 mg/day oral administration. Hydrocortisone 100 mg IV stat and repeat (in status asthmaticus). Budesonide or fluticasone are potent topical steroids that are used in asthma.

Miscellaneous agents

Antihistaminics and PAF antagonists offer svmptomatic relief by blocking receptors for respective mediators. Methotrexate and gold salts are supposed to modify course of the disease. Zileuton: Leukotrienes are the mediators of asthma. Lipooxygenase is the enzyme that is required for the synthesis of these LTs. Zileuton inhibits lipooxygenase and prevents attacks of asthma.

Line of management

Management usually started with intermitten sympathomimetic inhalors: Preferably β_2 selective agent, salbutamol. Alternatively oral β_2 stimulants also can be given

↓

If not controlled

↓

Add sodium cromoglycate or inhaled steroids.

↓

If not controlled

↓

High dose inhalational steroids or methyl xanthines or ipratropium bromide are added.

↓

If not controlled

Methyl xanthines + β stimulants + oral steroids or any suitable regimen that suits individual.

Steroids should be adjusted to minimum doses. Long term steroid therapy suppresses HPA axis and increases chances of superinfections due to immunosuppression. Short courses of tapering steroids are preferred to avoid withdrawal reactions.

Steroids should be adjusted to minimum doses.

Treatment of severe acute attack

Adrenaline 0.01 ml/kg or (0.2 - 0.5 ml of 1:1000) SC. Repeat after 30 minutes

Aminophylline - IV 250 mg in 10-20 ml normal saline over 10-15 minutes.

Salbutamol 100 mcg inhalation 2-3 times

Status asthmaticus

It is a medical emergency and should be treated immediately.

Immediate oxygen therapy

↓

Salbutamol oral or inhalational

↓

(CONT)

Prednisolone 30-60 mg oral or hydrocortisone 200 mg IV and repeat. In very severe conditions, aminophylline 250-500 mg in 20-50 ml of 5% glucose over half an hour.

Addition of ipratropium inhalation may improve refractory condition.

MANAGEMENT OF COUGH

Cough is a sudden expulsion of air from lungs. It is actually a protective reflex to prevent entry or existence of some foreign material into respiratory tract. Cough can be productive (attended with expectoration of material from bronchi) or nonproductive (dry). The material in productive cough needs to be removed of the tract. Hence, this is a useful cough. Nonproductive or dry cough is without expectoration and totally useless. Cough is a major symptom in almost all lower respiratory and some upper respiratory disorders. Some drugs like ACE inhibitors, levodopa, iodides, β blockers can induce cough.

Productive cough is useful cough.

Objectives of management of cough

i) To suppress cough

ii) To facilitate expulsion of secretions

Pharmacological management

Various drugs are used in the management of cough.

Figure 6.3 Drugs used in management of cough

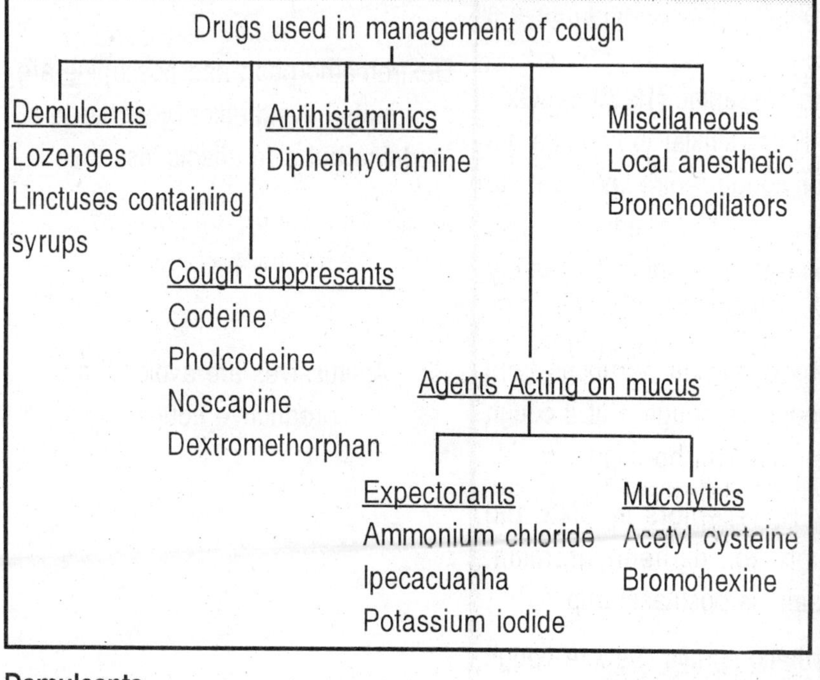

Demulcents

These agents have direct soothing effect on the mucosa of pharynx and trachea. They increase salivary secretion and create moist and warm atmosphere and prevent generation of impulses in respiratory tract (which stimulate cough centre). Lozenges or linctuses containing syrups are

Demulcents have direct soothing effect on the mucosa of pharynx and trachea.

act as demulcents. These are mainly useful in the cough originating from pharynx or upper part of trachea. For lower cough usually water arerosol inhalations with benzoin tincture is used. Menthol, due to aromatic properties, reduces stimulation of respiratory mucosa.

Mucokinetics

These agents increase water content of mucus and thus by reducing viscosity, facilitate removal of mucus and prevent irritation of respiratory mucosa. Potassium iodide, ipecac, guiphenesin are mucokinetics. Increase in respiratory secretions caused by these agents covers and protects irritated mucosa. This advantage makes these drugs useful in useless or dry cough.

Mucolytics

These agents break mucus and reduce viscosity of it liquefied mucus is removed easily. Bromhexine, acetyl cysteine, carbocysteine and pancreatic dornase are mucolytics. Inhalation of water aerosoles also has got same action.

Mucokytics reduce viscosity of mucus.

The term expectorant sometime is used collectively for mucolytics and mucokinetics.

Opioid antitussives

Opioids suppress cough centre in medulla and reduce cough reflex. It has also got some action on higher centres. Codeine or pholcodeine are preferred opioids as they have got more selective action on cough centre and lesser actions on CNS and have less constipating effect. They also have less addiction potential. Dose: Codeine up to 5 mg in children and up to 30 mg in adults. But codein is not useful in severe cough.

Dextromethorphan (10-20 mg QID oral) and noscapine (15-30 mg QID) are agents from the same class having efficacy similar to codeine but side effects less than it. These agents act on cough centre and increase its cough threshold for stimuli from respiratory tract and reduce cough. They have almost equal effectivity compared to opioids but safety profile is much better.

Dextromethorphan and noscapine are agents having efficacy similar to codeine but side effects less than it.

Antitussives, by suppressing cough, inhibit expulsion of mucus from respiratory tract, hence are avoided in productive cough. But if cough suppression is essential (even productive) they can be used.

Antitussives are avoided in productive cough.

Antihistaminics: Antihistamincs block H_1 receptors in CNS and produce sedation, which reduces cough. Ex. diphenhydramine, promethazine, etc. They are especially useful in postnasal drip.

Intractable cough responds to local anesthetic sprays. Severe cough sometimes demand bronchodilators. But use of both these agents in cough is controversial.

Intractable cough responds to local anesthetic sprays.

Management line

Figure 6.4 Management of cough

- Cough
  - Non productive
    - ↓ Cough suppressants (nonopioid or opioid)
  - Productive cough
    - Mucolytics
    - Mucolytics + antitussives

Antitussives are sometimes used even in productive cough:
i) Patient exhausted with cough
ii) Respiratory mucosal injuries
iii) Eye surgery

Lozenges (for upper respiratory cough) and water aerosol inhalations (for lower respiratory cough) are effective in all type of coughs. Lignocaine or bronchodilators are used in resistant cough.

Antibiotics are used in respiratory infections as curative treatment of cough.

MANAGEMENT OF POISONING

Almost any substance is capable of causing damage to body. Poisons are substance which, in relatively small amounts, may cause structural damage or functional disturbances in the body. Poisoning can be intentional (homicide or suicide) or accidental. Immediate treatment of the patient is crucial.

Absorption of oral poison is prevented by gastric lavage, by inducing vomiting, by using adsorbants or by bowel irrigation.

Objectives of management

i) Immediate care of deteriorating body functions
ii) Prevention of further absorption
iii) Promoting elimination of poison that is absorbed
iv) Specific antidotes for poisons.

I) Immediate care of deteriorating systems

Though it depends on the condition of the patient, certain measures that are commonly required in cases of poisonings are :

i) Keeping airway patent
ii) Endotracheal intubation
iii) Oxygen supply
iv) Fluid and electrolyte maintenance
v) Management of shock
vi) Antiarrhythmics, anticonvulsants, etc.

II) Prevention of further absorption

1) If poisoning is through skin or inhalation, patient must be shifted from that atmosphere immediately to avoid further exposure to poison.

2) Gastric lavage

In case poisoning is by oral route, poison in GI tract that is not absorbed, is removed by gastric lavage with warm water or saline. Some antidotes also can be introduced with gastric lavage. Gastric lavage is best effective in first four hours but can be effective over 24 hours depending on the rate of absorption of poison from GIT. Before giving lavage gag reflex must be checked, if it is not present endotracheal intubation is done prior to gastric lavage. Aspiration is a common problem with gastric lavage. In case of poisoning with corrosives or petroleum distillates, lavage is not done to avoid GI erosion and aspiration.

Gastric lavage is best effective in first four hours

In case of poisoning with corrosives or petroleum distillates, lavage is not done to avoid GI erosion and aspiration.

3) Emesis

Artificially induced vomiting also eliminates poison from GI tract. Emesis is induced with finger or spoon or ipecac syrup. It is best effective in first 2 hours but can be done for up to 12 hours after consumption of poison. Emesis is induced only in patients with normal reflex. Risk of aspiration is common with emesis induction. Emesis is not induced in unconscious patients and in cases of poisoning with corrosives and petroleum distillates.

4) Adsorbents

Activated charcoal (10 - 40 gm in water) is administered orally. It adsorbs poison and reduces absorption. It is not co-administered with ipecac as it adsorbs ipecac and makes it ineffective or ipecac induced vomiting expels charcoal out of GI tract. Administration of charcoal is effective in almost all poisonings except iron, lithium and corrosives. These agents are not adsorbed by charcoal.

5) Bowel irrigation or forceful purgation removes unabsorbed poison from GI tract.

III) Promoting elimination of poison

i) Inducing diuresis: If urine is made acidic, alkaline drugs remain in ionized form and are not reabsorbed back into blood. Therefore in case of poisoning with alkaline substances, urine is made acidic (Ex. amphetamine) In the same way in case of acidic poisons, alkalinization of urine is done.

Alterations in pH of urine can increase elimination of poison.

ii) Dialysis:

Dialysis is usually done in severe cases of poisonings. Blood is circulated out side the body and through a semipermeable membrane. Poisons pass out of blood. Filtered blood is sent back into body. If major part of poison is protein bound or if it is not in the blood (distributed in various tissues) then dialysis is not useful.

Dialysis can't remove poison that is protein bound and distributed.

iii) Charcoal hemoperfusion

Blood is passed through charcoal column outside the body. Charcoal adsorbs the poison and blood is returned in the body. Protein bound fraction of drug in plasma is also removed along with free drug, but if drug is distributed all over the body then hemoperfusion is of no use.

Charcoal hemoperfusion can't remove poison that is distributed.

iv) Peritoneal dialysis

External fluids are introduced in peritoneal cavity. Peritoneum acts as a semipermeable membrane and poison gets diffused into fluid. Fluid is then drained out. Peritoneal dialysis is not as effective as hemodialysis.

v) Activated charcoal to promote elimination

Poisons that are excreted through bile into GI tract can be reabsorbed back in the circulation. Repeated oral administration of charcoal prevents reabsorption of poison that is secreted in bile. This technique is effectively used in barbiturate or antidepressant poisonings.

Repeated oral administration of charcoal prevents reabsorption of poison that is secreted in bile.

IV) Specific measures for drug overdoses

Specific antidotes inhibit effects of poisons. Discussed here are roles of some antidotes in case of poisoning by different substances.

1) Overdose of anticoagulants: Antidote-Vit K. It replenishes the exhausted store of Vit K and promotes synthesis of clotting factor. (Refer Page 163).

2) Overdose of benzodiazepines: Antidote: flumazenil. Flumazenil competitively displaces benzodiazepines from benzodiazepine receptors and terminates their action.

3) Overdose of opioids: naloxone is opioid antagonist that prevents binding of opioids to opioid receptors.

4) Paracetamol poisoning: Effects of paracetamol poisoning are mainly due to toxic metabolites of paracetamol. Acetylcysteine, an antidote for paracetamol, replenishes enzyme glutathione, which inactivates toxic metabolites.

5) Digitalis poisoning: Digoxin specific antibody fragments are administered after digitalis poisoning. The antibodies form complexes with free digitalis, which are eliminated. (Refer page 149).

6) Salicylate poisoning: There is no specific antidote for it but force alkaline diuresis (frusemide with sodium bicarbonate) is crucial along with situational measures.

Poisonings by agonists of various receptors are usually treated by blockers of those receptors and vice versa. (certain measures are discussed in respective chapters).

Air pollutants

Environmental pollution is a growing problem of urbanization. Varieties of air pollutants have local and systemic toxic effects.

Air pollutants: Carbon monoxide
Nitrogen oxides
Sulphur dioxide
Hydrocarbons
Ozone

Air pollutants cause local and systemic toxicity.

Carbon monoxide poisoning

CO contributes almost half of the air pollutants. The sources of poisoning are charcoal fires, blast furnaces, gas engines or diesel engines. CO, after its entry into the body, combines with Hb and forms carboxyHb. It has a less oxygen carrying capacity.

Symptoms:

Throbbing headache, muscular weakness, nausea, vomiting, syncope, collapse, convulsions, cerebral edema, unconsciousness and coma. Death occurs usually due to respiratory arrest.

Management:

Fresh air

Pure and hyperbaric oxygen

Blood transfusion

Nikethamide: It stimulates respiratory centre. Rarely used drug.

Dexamethasone: (16-32 mg IV) in divided doses.

Diazepam: (5-10 mg IV) for convulsions.

Ozone poisoning

Ozone produces free radicals that cause oxidative damage and produce pulmonary irritation, edema and death. Symptomatic management is done in acute poisoning. A chronic exposure produces bronchitis, pulmonary fibrosis, hyperresponsiveness to antigens, etc. Antioxidants are used to avoid chronic toxicity. Nitrogen dioxide cause similar type of damage.

Petroleum products, cleaners, crude oils contain hazardous organic solvents: hydrocarbons. They are also capable of polluting air. Ex. Methane, benzene, ethane, carbon tetrachloride. They cause respiratory damage, carcinogenic changes, CNS depression, blood disorders.

Heavy metal poisoning and chelating agents

Heavy metals have astringent, caustic and bactericidal properties, but these agents have no therapeutic importance. They have toxicological significance. Heavy metals accumulate in the blood and cause toxicity, predominantly in liver, kidney, bone marrow, GI tract, nervous system, etc. Ex. Lead, arsenic, mercury, copper, gold, cadmium, antimony etc.

The mechanism for toxicity is their ability to form complexes with important biological radicals like sulfhydryl, hydroxy, carboxy, etc. This complex formation results in inhibition of enzymes containing that group. The lack of activity of that enzyme produces toxic effects.

Heavy metals form complexes with important biological radicals

Chelating agents

Chelating agents combine with metallic ions to form nontoxic, water-soluble complexes that are easily eliminated. Therefore these agents are used in heavy metal poisoning. Chelating agents that are used in clinical practice are: EDTA (Ethylene diamine tetra acetic acid)

Chelating agents combine with metallic ions to form nontoxic, water-soluble complexes that are easily eliminated.

dimercaprol, penicillamine, desferrioxamine, succimer, etc.

Sodium calcium edetate

This is a sodium calcium salt of edetate. It forms water-soluble nontoxic complexes with divalent and tetravalent metallic ions. It is not absorbed from GI tract and is given by injectable route.

Sodium calcium edetate is not absorbed from GI tract and is given by injectable route.

Indications

i) Diagnosis of lead poiconing

Sodium calcium edetate is administered intramuscularly (75 mg/kg) in 3 divided doses. If lead excretion in urine is more than 500 mg over next 24 hours, lead poisoning is confirmed.

ii) Treatment of lead poisoning

Injection of sodium calcium edetate is available in 200 mg/ml strength. It is diluted in 5% dextrose or 0.9% normal saline and administered by IV drip over 1 hour or by IM route in dose of 30-50 mg/kg/day in 2 divided doses for 5 days. Second similar course of 5 days is administered, if required. Total amount in course should not exceed 500 mg/kg

iii) It is rarely used in iron or cadmium poisoning.

Adverse effects: Renal impairment, thrombophlebitis, hypocalcemic tetany, febrile reactions, nausea, diarrhea, etc.

Disodium edetate: It is very much similar to sodium calcium edetate except for the fact that it has got affinity for calcium and it is used in hypercalcemia.

Dimercaprol: (British Anti Lewisite)

It is a chelating agent with a sulfhydryl groups. It forms nontoxic water soluble complexes with gold, antimony, arsenic, etc. It, not only prevents heavy metal induced inhibition of the enzymes but also reactivates them. Only problem with this agent is that the complexes formed by them are dissociable and metal ions get dissociated from complexes. To overcome this, the drug is administered in a dose which provides some free drug in excess. The excess drug forms complexes with the dissociated fraction of the metals.

Dimercaprol reactivates enzymes

Dimercaprol is administered in a dose which provides some free drug in excess.

Indications

i) Arsenic, mercury, gold, antimony poisoning.

Dose: Arsenic poisoning: 3 mg/kg IM every 4 hours.

Mercury poisoning: 5 mg/kg IM followed by 2.5 mg/kg IM BD for 10 days.

Lead poisoning: 4 mg/kg IM every 4 hours for 2 days and then every 6 hours for 2 days and then every 12 hours for 7 days. It can be used in combination with Ca Na edetate in lead poisoning.

2) Wilson's disease: Dimercaprol is used in this condition when penicillamine is contraindicated. (Refer page 236). Dose: 2.5 mg/kg/day

Adverse effects: tachycardia, rise in blood pressure, nausea, vomiting, headache, burning sensation in oral cavity, sweating, abscess at the site of injection, etc.

Penicillamine

It forms nontoxic water soluble complexes with copper, mercury, lead, etc. It can be given by oral route.

Penicillamine can be given by oral route

Indications:

i) Wilson's disease: This hepatolenticular degeneration disorder is characterized by abnormal copper metabolism and copper deposition predominantly in liver and brain. This results in degenerative changes in basal ganglia and liver cirrhosis. Penicillamine is a drug of choice in this condition. Dose: 1-5 gm/day, in divided doses, depending on the condition. Treatment is supported by copper deficient diet.

ii) Penicillamine is used in copper, mercury and lead poisoning. (500-1500 mg /day in 4 divided doses).

iii) Uses other than metallic disorders:

Rheumatoid arthritis: It causes reduction in IgM rheumatoid factor and suppresses the disease. It is also used in scleroderma and biliary disorders due to its immunological properties. (Dose 125-750 mg/day).

Desferrioxamine

It binds ferric ions to form nontoxic water-soluble complexes that are excreted in urine and bile. It also removes iron from hemosiderin.

Indications

i) Acute iron poisoning: Gastric lavage of desferrioxamine (2 g/l) is used as immediate treatment. Dose: 1 gm immediately, followed by 500 mg every 4 hours for 2 doses. Then 500 mg every 4-12 hours. Maximum amount should not exceed 6 gm in 24 hours. If patient is in a shock, 15 mg/kg/hr is used intravenously.

ii) In chronic iron intoxication 0.5 to 1 gm is used by IM route or 1-2 gm by SC route.

Management of lead poisoning

Poisoning with lead is usually by oral, respiratory or cutaneous routes. Water retained in lead pipes, inhalation of fumes from burning of batteries, lead painted toys, inhalation of fumes in glass or paint industries, lead added petrol are the common sources of lead poisoning. Lead is accumulated in erythrocytes, liver, kidney, bone, etc. Acute poisoning is rare.

Symptoms of acute poisoning

Metallic taste, cramp, black stools, shock, weakness, hemolytic crisis, etc.

Treatment of acute poisoning

Gastric lavage

Laxatives

Antispasmodics

Management of shock

Fluid replacement

Calcium disodium edetate (Refer page 235).

Barbiturate or mannitol as per requirement.

Chronic lead poisoning

Chronic lead poisoning is done over a prolonged period. It is observed in children playing with lead toys or in workers of printing or petroleum industries.

Symptoms of chronic lead poisoning

Metallic taste, cramps, constipation, black-blue line on gingival margins, (lead line), muscles weakness (lead palsy), microcytic hypochromic anemia, punctate basophilic stippling of erythrocytes, restlessness, irritability, headache, delirium, epilepsy (lead encephalopathy).

Treatment of chronic lead poisoning

Sodium calcium edetate (Refer page 235).

Succimer is another chelating agent that can be used as an alternative to edetate. Rarely penicillamine is used.

Symptomatic treatment includes: anticonvulsants, antispasmodics or mannitol (to reduce intracranial tension).

Mercury poisoning

Environmental pollution is the source of mercury poisoning. Workers in electrical industries or those in manufacturing units of thermometer, barometer are prone for this poisoning.

Symptoms of acute mercury poisoning

Choking, burning pain in stomach, white coating on tongue, hematuria, albuminuria, convulsions, metallic taste, collapse, gingival inflammation, arrhythmias, etc.

Treatment of acute poisoning

i) Charcoal, milk or egg to prevent further absorption

ii) Gastric lavage and respiratory support

iii) Fluid management: 5% glucose to induce diuresis

Dimercaprol (Refer page 235). 300 mg dimercaprol (deep IM) immediately, 150 mg BD for 2-3 days. Alternatively penicillamine is used.

Chronic poisoning

Contaminated fish diet is the source of chronic mercury poisoning.

Symptoms of chronic mercury poisoning

GI disturbances, excess salivation, swollen salivary glands, brown blue lines on gums, loose teeth, tremors of tongue and fingers.

Treatment

Oral hygiene

Prophylactic measures

Dimercaprol
Hemodialysis

Arsenic poisoning

Arsenic is found in well water, soil, air, etc. Smelting of copper or lead releases arsenic into environment. It is also used as herbicide or pesticide. It looks like sugar. It is cheap and easily available and commonly used for homicidal poisoning. Printing industry is also a common source of poisoning.

Acute arsenic poisoning

Though it is rare, a specific form of arsenic (AS_2O_3) that is readily available and has appearance of sugar, is responsible for acute poisoning. It leads to GI discomfort, burning lips, difficulty in swallowing, salivation, vomiting, diarrhea, cramps, convulsion, visual disturbances etc.

Treatment

Gastric lavage
Emetics
Large amount of water mixed with freshly prepared hydrated ferric oxide is introduced in stomach. It converts arsenious acid in non toxic formic arsenite. Dimercaprol 2.5-3 mg/kg 4 hrly for 2 days and 6-8 hrly for 10 days or penicillamine one week with meals is the treatment of choice.

Symptoms of chronic arsenic poisoning

Lack of appetite
Muscle weakness
Skin pigmentation of neck
Brittle nail
Garlic odor to breath
Jaundice, anemia
Peripheral neuropathy
Nephropathy

Treatment

Long term antidotes or supportive measures are required

Cyanide poisoning

Accidental inhalation of hydrocyanic acid, ingestion of nitroprusside, bitter almonds, fumigations in industries are common sources of cyanide poisoning. Cyanide reacts with cytochrome oxidase in mitochondria. This inhibits cellular respiration which results in histotoxic anoxia, cellular dysfunction and death within minutes of inhalation. Inhalational poisoning is instant.

Symptoms: Headache, dizziness, drowsiness, dyspnea, convulsions, coma, death.

Treatment: Gastric lavage is essential in case of poisoning by oral route. Diagnosis is usually made by typical odor. Amyl nitrite inhalation 0.2 ml every 2 minutes or IV sodium nitrite 10 ml of 3% IV is administered immediately. Nitrates produce less toxic metabolites: methhemoglobin (Refer Page 145). As cobalt has affinity for cyanide dicobalt edetate is also used in cyanide poisoning. Sodium thiosulphate (50 ml of 25% IV over 20 minutes) accelerates detoxification of cyanides.

Methanol poisoning

Methanol is a cheap substitute for ethyl alcohol. It follows zero order kinetic (Refer page 24).It accumulates in the body and causes variety of adverse effects including blindness, acidosis and coma. Methanol, during its metabolism in the body, gets converted into formaldehyde and formic acid with the help of enzymes alcohol dehydrogenase and aldehyde dehydrogenases. These metabolites are responsible for toxicity. Ethyl alcohol is an antidote in methanol poisoning. Ethyl alcohol utilizes same enzymes for its metabolism and prevents formation of toxic metabolites from methanol. Metabolites of ethyl alcohol are nontoxic. 50% oral solution of ethyl alcohol (1 mg/kg) or 5% ethyl alcohol in 5% dextrose IV is used for this purpose. Sodium bicarbonate is used if metabolic acidosis is present.

Poisoning due to herbicides or pesticides

These are some of the agents that are responsible for poisoning.

1) Anticholinesterase poisoning (OP poisoning): (Refer page 77).

2) Parquet poisoning: It is a weed killer herbicide and is highly poisonous. (even 10 ml can be fatal) Now most of the parquet formulations are made bad odored and emetics are added to it to prevent poisoning. Burning sensations, GI ulceration and alveolitis leading to pulmonary edema are the consequences of poisoning. Death is usually due to respiratory or renal failure. Cleaning of skin and eyes is important. Intraocular antibiotics are used to prevent infections. Lavage with Fuller's earth (aluminium silicate), forced alkaline diuresis, mannitol (to reduce edema), hemodialysis are different ways of management of these patients.

Dinitro compound poisoning

These are insecticides and herbicides and are absorbed from the skin. Yellow staining, tachycardia, deep breathing convulsions and coma are the consequences of dinitro poisoning. Fluid and electrolyte balance is crucial. They must be distinguished from OP poisoning (as in dinitro poisoning atropine is contraindicated).

☆ ☆ ☆